Pandemic A Call to Love

By Rose Bruce, EdD, PhD

Maple Leaf Publishing Inc.
Alberta Canada

Pandemic A Call to Love
Copyright © 2020 by Rose B.

All rights reserved. No part of this book may be reproduced or transmitted in any form or by any means, electronic or mechanical, including photocopying, recording, or by any information storage and retrieval system, without written permission of the publisher.

ISBN Paperback: 978-1-77419-047-0
ISBN eBook: 978-1-77419-048-7
Rev. Date: June 8, 2020

MAPLE LEAF PUBLISHING INC.

3rd Floor 4915 54 St Red Deer,
Alberta T4N 2G7 Canada

General Inquiries & Customer Service
Phone: 1-(403)-356-0255
Toll Free: 1-(888)-498-9380
Email: info@mapleleafpublishinginc.com

Other Books by Dr. Rose Bruce

A Layperson's Guide to Understanding Research and Data Analysis, Lynda Rose Bruce, EdD, PhD, 2013, Xlibris LLC.

My Spiritual Unfolding: Science of Mind,
Rose Bruce, EdD, PhD, 2020, Maple Leaf Publishing

Foreword

During the Covid-19 pandemic many of us have read with interest how people coped with the 1918 influenza pandemic a century ago. And we are grateful that people back then took the time to chronicle their thoughts, feelings, and impressions. Reading these past accounts make us feel less alone in the universe. Similarly, a century from now people will appreciate reading Dr. Rose Bruce's account of this cataclysmic event that has undoubtedly marked our twenty-first century, just like the World Wars and the 1920's Great Depression in the twentieth century, characterize the previous century.

Written for the future, Pandemic: A Call to Love, is also useful for all of us today. It is an intimate conversation, a sharing of our personal feelings about the trials and tribulations we face day to day. As Dr. Bruce puts it, "it sheds some light into the darkness of these times."

Her narrative evokes the kind of writing that is done by someone who is in the frontline trenches of a war, someone who is under a barrage of fire. The reader can feel the tension of dealing with an invisible threat that forces us to be "sheltered-at-home" or else risk losing our lives or the lives of others. This experience is also akin to culture shock, because our everyday routines, habits, sights, interactions, are no longer there. Our world has shrunk to the space of our home and the occasional trips to the grocery store. Under such conditions, a writer must, appropriately, focus on writing down impressions rather than following academic formalities. As Dr. Bruce states, "One of the reasons I left academia was because I was so tired of just relying on the mind and ignoring the heart. "

I met Dr. Bruce at Sonoma State University when I first got there thirty years ago, and I can attest that the academic separation of what in Buddhism is known as "the heart-mind" weighs heavily on a person.

Dr. Bruce has always manifested loving kindness to all of us who had the pleasure of interacting with her in her position as Director of Testing to the Associate Vice President of Institutional Research, as well as professor, colleague, and friend.

We cannot, alas, ignore academic analysis. As a professor of the History of Ideas, Literature and Philosophy for four decades, I find Dr. Bruce's book is more than just a description of events on a given day. It is a modernist work, more akin to James Joyce's' stream-of-consciousness than to a journal because it illustrates an existential phenomenon: how Content overcomes Form. What I mean by this is that in her Prelude, she states, "Each chapter starts with the Daily Thought from Beyond 20/20 Spiritual Vision by the Center for Spiritual Living in Santa Rosa, California." Yet, the intense reality of these times overwhelms this plan and, to the reader's delight, the content encompasses much more than the Covid-19 epidemic. It includes book reviews, biographical sketches, charts, and web links. This is not unintentional. As she herself notes: "The thoughts did not easily translate into what was happening around me…." I find that this to be an enrichment of her personal account.

Furthermore, rather than provide a description of "the practice of everyday life" in which we appropriate news and social media to mold it according to our own individual experience (Michel de Certeau), Dr. Bruce presents what Parker Palmer advices in his book by the same name: Let Your Life Speak. In this sense, it is also Postmodernist work. To the Postmodernist question, "Who speaks?", Dr. Bruce has two answers: Life speaks, life imposes itself, and ultimately, Love speaks.

Dr. Bruce's account is centered on the notion of the symbiotic and loving, spiritual interrelationship of all sentient beings in the world. This ancient knowledge is in constant struggle with the egotistic, survival-of-the-fittest claim that we are instead self-sufficient individuals that should either learn to survive on our own or simply, in its more extreme versions, just die.

Dr. Bruce illustrates this struggle when she notes the efforts to assist people on the one hand, and the lack of positive leadership of the Government of the United States to provide the necessary resources and equipment to fight the virus. Some of our elected officials even argue that saving the economy is more important than saving lives, that this is Mother Nature's way of "thinning the herd."

These are dangerous times for the concept of what it is to be human, to be humane. The notion of "thinning the herd" does not take into consideration the realities of income inequality. On the one hand, low-income people who lack access to good nutrition, and health maintenance as well as knowledge about these subjects, are the ones who are more prone to infection and death. Proportionally, this means that Blacks, Native Americans, and Latinos are the primary victims of this disease. Nevertheless, the armed protestors that Dr. Bruce mentions, demand the end of sheltering at home and the opening of business which, inevitably, will lead to an increase Covid-19 cases. Yet it is not only racism that is at play. Covid-19 also targets the elderly and people who are immune-suppressed. These people are also considered by some as being dispensable, or part of God's plan to "clean the barn." These claims echo the Nazi policy of getting rid of "undesirable" people who did not fit the model of the superior race.

These are, to be sure, desperate times when people's livelihood, their very survival, is threatened, and in such times many people lose their sense of humanity and interconnection. Dr. Bruce is not one of them. On the contrary, her voice echoes, W.H. Auden's words: "We must love one another or die." Dr. Bruce chronicles, many people from diverse ethnicity and social class who, lovingly, step up to volunteer and carry on the basic functions of society. These are the nurses, doctors, grocery employees, deliverers, etc. While reading her book, one not only follows but feels the ebb and flow of emotions as days and then weeks go by punctuated with alternating good news and bad news, spiritual epiphanies, and exasperation. Just as the spring comes after the winter, however, she finds constant rejuvenation in spiritual readings, meditation and prayers.

And this is precisely why her book is a call to love and an inspiration to us today and to our future descendants.

>Francisco H. Vázquez, Ph.D.
>Windsor, California May 16, 2020

Contents

Foreword..2-3-4-5
Prelude..8

The Pandemic Starts
Saturday, March 21, 2020..9
Tuesday, March 24, 2020..............................10-11-12-13
Wednesday, March 25, 2020....................................14-15
Friday, March 27, 2020..16-17-18

Spokesperson Script for
My Spiritual Unfolding: Science of Mind................19-20

Saturday, March 28, 2020..21-22

Lynda Rose Bruce
Autobiography 23-24-25-26-27

Endangered Species Directory.............................27-28-29-30

Sunday, March 29, 2020..31-32-33
Monday, March 30, 2020........................34-35-36-37-38-39
Tuesday, March 31, 2020...40-41
Wednesday, April 1, 2020..........................42-43-44-45-46
Friday, April 3, 2020.................................47-48-49-50-51-52
Palm Sunday, April 5, 2020......................................53-54-55
Monday, April 6, 2020..56-57-58
Tuesday, April 7, 2020..59-60
Wednesday, April 8, 2020.......................................61-62-63
Thursday, April 9, 2020..64
Good Friday, April 10, 2020...65

What is Trement?..66-67-68-69

Saturday, April 11, 2011..70-71
Easter Sunday, April 12, 2020..72-73
Monday, April 13, 2020..74
Tuesday, April 14, 2020...75-76
Wednesday, April 15, 2020..77-78
Thursday, April 16, 2020..79-80
Tuesday, April 28, 2020..81-82-83
May 12, 2020..84-85
Wednesday, May 13, 2020...86-87-88-89

Prelude

This is a deeply personal account of my experience of the Covid-19 pandemic impacting the United States in 2020. I am a spiritual person and try to bring a spiritual perspective to all of life's events. I continued to do this with the pandemic. Each chapter starts with the Daily Thought from Beyond 20/20 Spiritual Vision by the Center for Spiritual Living in Santa Rosa, California. I start each day reading this as a way to frame the events of the day. The thoughts did not easily translate into what was happening around me, but it did help ground me in a spiritual response to the fear that was so evident in our society during this time.

It is meant as one person's account not necessarily representative of the general population. However, I share this journal so that, years from now, when this has all been forgotten, there will be a story of my coping. I hope that it sheds some light into the darkness of these times.

Sincerely,

Rose Bruce

The Pandemic Starts
Saturday, March 21, 2020

"I let go and see the evidence of Love in action all around me. The love of the Divine inspires me to express my love for self, others, and for life itself."

The pandemic of the Covid-19 virus is hitting the United States and the world. It started in Wuhan China in late December 2019 and has gradually spread throughout the world in spite of entire cities in China to shut down requiring that their residents say indoors. Passengers on cruise ships and airplanes have spread it in spite of quarantining passengers for two weeks in precaution of spreading it. It is causing great fear but it is also calling out great love and reassurance. People are needing each other as never before and are reaching out in humility and need. Our hearts are opening.

I just read in Love Without End: Jesus Speaks by Glenda Green Jesus that there is currently great love being sent to the earth and with it will come a collapse of structures which have held our society together before. This destruction is necessary to usher in a new era of love, sisterhood and brotherhood as has never been seen before on this earth. It is a time for unity.

Each moment we have a choice to be in love or in fear. Fear is not the opposite of love but rather is an alternative to love. Love is all that exists, but we fail to see that when we choose other realities such as fear or greed. Our work is to discard the illusion of separateness and choose love and unity. We are each an individualized expression of the Divine here to make our own unique contribution. Through meditation and prayer, we can strengthen our connection with the Divine and discern how best to express the love that we are. This is a sacred time.

Tuesday, March 24, 2020

"NEWNESS – Today, I give up the idea that I can repeat anything. Creative Mind within me reveals itself as newness in my thoughts, words, and creativity. This creativity flows out from me and is a blessing to all who come into contact with it."

We are truly living in amazing times! Today I learned from the World Health Organization (WHO) that it took 60 days for the first 100,000 cases of Covid-19 to develop, that number was added in the next 11 days to 200,000 and in the last four days it has gone to 300,000 cases worldwide. We are experiencing a time of either fear or love. States in the U.S. are having to outbid each other to purchase testing kits for the coronavirus from $4 a kit to $6 a kit. Protective gear for hospital staff is in short supply and people are being advised to only wear a mask if you have the virus and let hospital workers have the safety gear to take care of patients. Personal Protective Gear (PPE) includes an N-95 face mask, plastic face covering, goggles, plastic gloves, plastic gown covering the entire body, and plastic foot coverings. There are pictures of doctors and nurses lifting off their face masks after a long shift with indentations where the device suctioned to their face. They must try to protect themselves from getting the virus. Some are successful, other are not. Spaces are being created to hold hospital beds outside of the hospitals as they will be overrun with need. The navy has sent the ship USS Mercy to New York and USS Comfort to San Francisco to help. They can take non-virus patients such as trauma patients freeing up much needed beds in stateside hospitals.

People are continuing to be asked to stay inside for the safety of all. Most people in my area in Northern California are staying inside. I am still walking around Spring Lake everyday staying three to six feet away from other people walking. We are not allowed to be in gatherings of more than ten people. All restaurants and bars, schools, churches and gyms are closed until further notice. Large gatherings of any kind have been cancelled: professional sporting events, concerts, the Olympics in Tokyo et cetera. Young people in their 20s and 30s are not paying attention to the warnings thinking that they are immune from infection but that is not the case.

In the U.S. people are hoarding toilet paper. On the TV are images of people with shopping carts full of toilet paper. I guess that is what they can get their heads wrapped around at this unusual time.

It is a time to think about others above self. We need to stay inside or at a safe distance from others so that we do not spread the disease faster. At the end of the news cast this evening there were shots of people calling in on their cell phones singing John Lennon's song Imagine "imagine all the people, living for today…" We are now experiencing that reality.

The World Health Organization yesterday called upon the world to stop all acts of was as we are at war against the virus and must come together for the common good. U.S. Military in Afghanistan and other foreign countries are being recalled to protect them from the virus.

I can go out to get food or medicine but must be very careful. Wearing disposable plastic gloves is recommended while shopping and all packages must be sprayed with nine parts water and one-part alcohol to disinfect.

Eric needs to take his mom to an appointment with the surgeon tomorrow. It has been scheduled for a month and she needs to see him because her hip surgery went wrong and she needs corrective surgery. She is in increasing pain. Hopefully she will be able to get treatment soon. We shall see.

The stock market has dropped from a high of 28,000 to 18,000 points. It will lead to a recession worse than the 2008 real estate recession. Investors are waiting to hear if Congress passes a one trillion dollar stimulus bill to bail out large and big business (airplanes, tourism, travel, restaurants, small business owners et cetera) and people ($1,200 per adult stimulus to pay rent and buy food). We need the country to come together but it is not doing so far.

How am I coping? I only allow myself one hour of news a day: the PBS Newshour. CNN is running continuous coverage of the coronavirus pandemic. It would be easy to be overwhelmed with fear if one watched it all day. I go for my morning walks then come home and eat lunch. When the word first came out on the news we went to Costco and bought a month's worth of food, so we are safe in that regard. I have my retirement income and we both have social security so our finances are secure. I have been getting exciting emails about my first and second books (The Gift of Sobriety: A Spiritual Transformation and My Spiritual Unfolding: Science of Mind). I now have confirmed film rights to the first book in English and French. I have a NETFLIX offer on my second book. Translation rights of the first and second book in Spanish, Arabic, French and French Canadian have also been secured. So, I am quite busy taking care of business, writing a trailer and video script for the second book, and now writing this third book. I love my life and feel very blessed. I have over 20,000 followers on my author Facebook page at Rosesobriety.com. I post something each Friday or Saturday, something positive and thoughtful prompted by my readings. My class at the Center for Spiritual Living in Santa Rosa, California just ended so I am disciplining myself to keep reading spiritual books. I use Zoom to have recovery meetings online. I saw my counselor online but that didn't go as well as usual. It is hard to feel the energetic connection over the internet.

I am meditating on the phrase "They Grace is my sufficiency" from Joel Goldsmith's book Practicing the Presence. I find it gives me great comfort.

In short, I am living my life as normally as possible. Spiritual fitness takes effort just like physical health takes effort. Habits can either save us or sink us.

In just one day the number of cases of Covid-19 worldwide has jumped another 100,000 to 407,000+ cases with 18,227 deaths. In the United States today we have 50,000 cases with 646 deaths.

It is estimated that the numbers could keep escalating at this rapid rate for weeks or months. This is in spite of people staying home from work and away from social gatherings. Jails nationwide are releasing nonviolent inmates by as much as 25% of the total population in order to stop the spread of the virus in that population. In New York, the fastest growing city with cases in the U.S. today, cases are doubling every night.

The response by the Federal government has been less than satisfactory. President Trump has consistently given out misinformation in hopes of getting people to go back to work to stimulate the economy. News casters have to correct what misinformation he has provided. It is a dangerous situation and people have died because he gave out false information about a malaria drug that "might" work but in fact has been killing people with the virus. Hopefully he will be voted out of office in November this year.

Wednesday, March 25, 2020

"HEALTH — Today, I give up the idea that there is anything in me other than a perfect light from God. The light of God resides in each cell of my physical being and is ready to respond to the love I shower on my body."

The park where I go to walk every morning was closed this morning. I went there as usual and the road to the parking lot was closed. I got out and started walking as usual and saw a sign restricting people from walking. Perhaps tomorrow I will go and walk anyway.

I then went to the grocery store and saw that they were letting in people one at a time. There was a line outside the store with people standing three feet apart that was a block long. I left my cart and walked away.

I then went to Target to get some medicine that needed to be picked up. I roamed the grocery area for food and the shelves were empty. I was able to get the last two packages of carrots, the last package of celery, some peppers for omelets, and the last two packages of butter. It is very odd and worrisome. I came home and fixed a tri tip roast that Eric had defrosted with cooked carrots and cheese filled pasta. It felt normal and reassuring.

The news is all about the Covid-19 pandemic. India has now ordered all 1.3 billion residents to stay inside. This is already the case in the U.S., Canada, South Korea, Italy, Spain, France, the UK and Iran. In the U.S. there are 64,800 cases with 971 deaths. Hospitals are started to fill up. The hardest hit states are New York, California, Washington, Oregon and Louisiana (after they allowed the Mardi Gras to occur this week). The Congress and House signed a three trillion-dollar rescue package for the nation. But it is said that the money will not get to residents on unemployment insurance until May. Landlords are not allowed to have evictions now and mortgages can go unpaid for a while. The main priority is medical supplies for people on the frontline of this:

doctors, nurses, custodians and technicians. There are not enough test kits and protective gear to meet the need.

Today I learned that a friend has the virus. She sent an email. I told her how sorry I was and to keep in touch. She has respiratory problems so she is very vulnerable to the virus. It attacks the lungs first. I pray for her.

I am using discipline to NOT get totally caught up in news of the virus. I am watching a series on TV, The Affair, that is free during the next three weeks. Everyone is doing their part to help. I tried to pay some bills online and saw a notice that their server and other bank's servers had been hacked. Personal identification including credit cards, social security numbers, names and address had been compromised.

I received an email from Ed McPherson on the requirements to get my second book qualified for a NETFLIX series. He already has the funding for it. I contacted Maple Leaf Publishing to get the necessary trailer and video hits paid for. I was told they are shutting down for three weeks starting tomorrow. The BookExpo scheduled for the end of May in New York has been postponed until the end of July. I will go back and sign film, book translation, and NETFLIX contracts then, God willing.

I am writing the book, which helps. Eric came home this morning after taking care of his mom an hour and a half away and that helps, just having him around helps me feel like things are somewhat normal.

How long can this last? I must double up on spiritual reading and meditation.

Friday, March 27, 2020

"Strength – Today, I give up the idea of weakness in favor of the idea of one, all-pervasive power permeating all of Creation. I call that power my strength."

I wonder if the pandemic is the earth fighting back? We have abused Mother Earth terribly. We have polluted her oceans with plastics. We have allowed CO_2 to be in the atmosphere because of automobiles and oil refineries to the point that the polar ice caps are melting. Endangered species are disappearing. I went online to query "endangered species photos" and found page after page of beautiful animals and birds. The coronavirus appears to have a mortality rate of 4%. It might help the earth a lot to lose four percent of its population.

Today there are 123,500+ new cases of Covid-19 in the U.S. with 8,600 reported deaths. The cases in the U.S. are the highest for any country with 78,600+ cases and 1,136 deaths. Italy has 900 deaths per day now. The health care system is maxed out and doctors are having to decide who gets a ventilator and who doesn't with older people being left to die. Prime Minister Johnson of Great Brittan has the virus now as does their Minister of Health. Newscasters on TV are reporting from their homes. To me it is reassuring seeing their homes instead of the sterile news rooms. Humanity is starting to come together in a common good. We are all in this together. Borders do not matter to the virus.

In the U.S. General Motors has been nationalized by the federal government to start making ventilators. There are 160,000 needed in New York according to Governor Cuomo and they have only 30,000. Health care workers in New York are protesting their working conditions. They are only given one face mask to last a week leaving them susceptible to infection. New Orleans has turned its convention center into a morgue to store all of the bodies. They held Mardi Gras in late February leaving many people open to infections. Symptoms do not show up for a week allowing transmission without our knowledge.

Wall Street continues to take deep dives with occurring increases. The Down Jones Industrial Average has swung from a high in the 28,000s to 18,000 the biggest swing since 1938. We are at war. At war against the virus. Today it is at 21,636 bouncing back after the relief package of two trillion dollars that the Congress passes yesterday and the President signed into law. It will give people on unemployment an additional $600. Last week 3.5 million people in the U.S. filed for unemployment.

Everyone in the U.S. and most of the world is ordered to stay at home. I have cleaned every surface of my house, waxed the floors, and reorganized the kitchen counters. Today Eric, my husband, is reorganizing the kitchen cabinets. I am making a stew in the crock pot with what produce and meat I could buy at the store: beef stew meat, celery, carrots, green beans, onion, a stew flavoring packet Eric bought and chicken bouillon as I am out of beef bouillon. When Eric was up in Lake County, an hour and a half North, taking care of him mom last week they had groceries. There is no more food on the shelves here. I sent him up with a long list to shop up there tomorrow when he returns to take care of his mom. She needs a hip replacement but when they went to the doctor's appointment, she was told the surgery had to be postponed for two to three months because of the virus. He is giving her 10mg of melatonin in the morning and evening to help her sleep and not be in so much pain. She has had fentanyl patches and hydromorphone pills for over ten years and they don't give her much relief anymore. Doctors have been cutting down on her pain pills because of the oxycodone overdoses the past few years.

The number of cases worldwide of Covid-19 has now reached 511,600+ with 23,500 dead. In the United States we have 78,600+ cases with 1,136 deaths. I cannot go a State park anymore for my daily walk because they are all closed. You can get a fine of $500 for going into the park and can even go to jail for it. I did not walk today.

I added the following Spiritual Mind Treatment that I wrote to the Facebook page on my website Rosesobriety.com.

If you are feeling anxious, read the following to yourself.

Unconditional Love is the basis of all that is: seen and unseen. It moves through the universes and through the smallest atom in perfect harmony. There is a natural rhythm to all things.

I know this Love is who I am. It expresses through me and as me.

I rejoice in this knowing and rest in the assurance that all is well. This Love guides me to be still and listen. It prompts me to move and speak when it is time. I need only rest in this Divine Love and all is well. Fear does not enter here. Only Light and Love abide. I am at peace. I am whole and complete. Nothing is lacking. I am upheld and supported by this Love. All is well.

I give thanks for this knowing, this shift in consciousness. I give thanks for this peace.

I release it knowing it is set into the Law of Life and is manifesting now as I speak.

And so it is.

I also finished the video script for my second book *My Spiritual Unfolding: Science of Mind.*

Spokesperson Script for
My Spiritual Unfolding: Science of Mind

By **Rose Bruce, EdD, PhD**

I would like to talk with you today about a remarkable book I read recently that concerns an issue of importance to many people today: spirituality in everyday living. Dr. Bruce brings to light her intimate understanding of deep spiritual transformation following a descent into alcoholism. One and a half years into recovery from alcohol addiction she sensed a deeper spiritual longing. She was led to attend the Center for Spiritual Living in Santa Rosa, California that teaches the concepts of Science of Mind or New Thought as described by Ernest Holmes, Emmet Fox, Emma Curtis Hopkins and others.

Dr. Bruce took classes consistently during the next fifteen months gaining a continually deepening understanding of the spiritual principles and their application to her life and the life of others. A part of the philosophy is a healing technique called Spiritual Mind Treatment. Dr. Bruce describes what this is, how it is done, and how she has applied it to many situations in her life. She translates sometimes complex concepts into simple behaviors, patterns of thought and meditative practices that can used by anyone no matter what their religious background may be.

Larry A. Burr from Cotati, California writes the following review.

My Spiritual Unfolding: Science of Mind beautifully expresses how the promises of peace and love manifest when an individual embraces the key to transformation – trust in spiritual guidance. It amazes me how much Rose has embraced her own spirituality and found it to be the foundation of not only sobriety but a good life. I feel her belief and trust through these stories, and I celebrate how spirituality is changing her life and filling it with peace and joy.

Rose's My Spiritual Unfolding: Science of Mind grips me due to the authenticity she expresses through her struggles. I love reading about the characters in her life and how her relationships change as her spirituality grows. I am inspired to know that it gets easier the more you practice spiritual concepts and that no one can do it perfectly. My Spiritual Unfolding: Science of Mind is a lovely balance between struggle and the process of change through spiritual conditioning.

The first thing I think about when I reflect on her books is how much I relate to story after story. Everyone's story is obviously different, and Rose has been able to express through her stories the emotional and mental core that everyone can relate to. Anyone wanting to get sober could use them as an indicator of what emotions, struggles and experiences they will likely encounter.

The book **My Spiritual Unfolding: Science of Mind** by Dr. Rose Bruce can be bought at Amazon, Barnes and Nobles, or from her website rosesobriety.com starting at the end of May 2020 . Her insights offer wisdom and guidance to people in similar situations. Her website rosesobriety.com is an excellent resource of her blog, reviews, trailers, articles, upcoming events and order information. Look for it today!

Saturday, March 28, 2020

"I let go and see the evidence of Love in action all around me. The love of the Divine inspires me to express my love for self, others, and for life itself."

I just got off a recovery meeting via Zoom. It is so reassuring to see the faces and hear the voices of my friends in recovery. People are talking about how hard it is to be isolated for so long. Eric and I have been indoors for three weeks now. Last week we were no longer allowed to go to public parks which had been a large part of my coping skills. It is too dangerous for people to be out now. You can get a ticket or a large fine if you don't have a good reason to leave you home.

Now more than ever it is a call to love to handle this situation. Many people are dropping into fear and that is the enemy now. I had a friend call and she was worried about how she will recover financially when this is over. I suggested she just focus on dealing with today. Jumping to fear of the future is only harmful at any time and especially now. The "one day at a time" philosophy of recovery serves us well now. Many in recovery don't like being isolated as that was such a big part of their addictive lifestyle.

I am starting to feel achy and tired. Fortunately, I went back to the pharmacy last week to get the only two boxes of ibuprofen left on the shelf. I need it today. I have one friend with the virus. It helps to keep this journal. I could never have imagined this scenario in my life and others in the future may have difficulty imagining it also. A daily log is the only way to capture the details that seem so obvious at the time but fade over time.

Eric has gone up to Lake County to take care of him mom Becky. He goes there at least two days a week. The caregiver for the other days failed to show up on Wednesday which was her responsibility. I am not sure why. I hope she can continue to take the other five days.

Fortunately, we have lots of meat in the freezer. We can go a long time without additional food. Eric bought me a cheesecake from the Cheesecake Factory which I am devouring at this time. It is reassuring to have this luxury in my life. It reminds me of old time of abundance. We have our wonderful home to be in with heat and food. We have nothing to complain about.

I just finished writing my autobiography for my application to the Certificate for Spiritual Education at the Holmes Institute. Life will go on and get back to normal. I plan to enter the program this September, 2020.

Lynda Rose Bruce
Autobiography

I was born September 18, 1949 into a Swedish Lutheran family in Kansas. I was the last of three daughters. The midwestern values of honesty, hard work, discipline, family, and academic excellence were instilled in me. Dad was a pilot during WW II then came home to work at Boeing building airplanes. He was transferred to Takoma, Washington and at age three I moved to the West Coast. Mom stayed home making a safe and welcoming place with traditional Swedish dishes and weekly church attendance. We moved to Takoma, Washington when I was three and to Oakland, California when I was 1fifteen.

I had been raised to be a wife and mother and married at nineteen as had my mother and two older sisters. I had two years of college under my belt and went to work to put my husband through college. All was going according to plan. Then one day I came home from work to find that my husband had removed all of his belongings from the home and withdrawn half of our checking and savings account. I was stunned. He finally called later that night to say he had moved out and wanted a divorce. My world shattered.

I eventually decided to travel in Mexico, Central and South America with a male friend I had met who had lived in Spain for two years. Thus, began seven months of adventure and introspection, studying Spanish and yoga as we went. I returned with a sense of responsibility to do something with my life.

I decided to attend California State University in Chico and moved there. For the next six years I studied psychology and counseling receiving a BA and MA respectively. I also studied Kodenkan Ju Jitsu and earned a Black Belt. I was finding myself. It was at that time that I decided to change my name to Rose. A new identity had emerged.

After graduating I was offered a job on campus as the Psychometrist in the Testing Office. I had loved learning statistics as a graduate student and felt right at home. I got married to a fellow employee at Tower Records, Gary, where I worked to put myself through college.

Gary got a job in Sonoma County and we moved there. I heard about an opening as a Psychometrist at Sonoma State University the day before the application period ended. I applied and got the job. My Higher Power had stepped in to guide me in a new direction. Thus, began a new period of stability lasting fourteen years. After two years at work my boss retired and I was offered his position on the condition that I earn a doctorate. I shopped around and finally decided on an EdD program at the University of California in Berkeley in quantitative methods in educational psychology. I loved it. I received my EdD in 1994.

Ten years into our marriage, while I was in the doctoral program, he was suddenly diagnosed with AIDS. It was the 1980s and AIDS was just starting to spread in the Bay Area and the world. I had thought he had the flu and was quite startled when I heard the diagnosis. The doctor looked at me as though I were dead when I said we had not practiced protective sex. Why would we? I was tested and was not infected. My Higher Power had again guided and protected me without my awareness. I had the decision to choose fear or love. I chose love and took care of him for the next three year and three months. He died peacefully in his sleep at home in our bed.

When Gary was diagnosed with AIDS, I read everything I could on healing, death and dying. I ran across a book by Caroline Myss in which she claimed to have healed a client of AIDS by helping him come to grips with his homosexuality. I was fascinated and began attending weekend workshops taught by her and Dr. Norm Shealy on energetic healing. I became interested in the mind-body relationship. This eventually led to me receiving my PhD from the school they founded Holos University for Graduate Seminary.

When Gary died, grief was again my lot. I struggled to get a new footing. Fortunately, I had my work to return to. Eventually I was ready to open my heart. I had for several years had a profound friendship with a woman, Leslie, whom I met in a statistics class I had taught at Sonoma State University. She was a lesbian. I felt safe and close to her. One day at lunch she was recounting with sadness memories about her mother's death and I reached out my hand to hold hers in comfort. This began my gradual acceptance of her as a lover and eventually life partner and wife. She had a BA with distinction in Mathematics and Master's in Psychology from Sonoma State and we had much in common. We could discuss any topic from spirituality to statistics to art. I was amazed when she moved in how many books we had in common.

I worked at Sonoma State University for thirty years in increasing capacity eventually becoming the Associate Vice President of Institutional Research. I retired at age 60 planning to spend many happy years with Leslie. After one year she was diagnosed with cancer. One year later she died on December 27, 2014.

Once again, I was in loss and grief. This time I had no work to occupy my mind and time. I gradually slipped into a deep depression exacerbated by alcohol abuse. I had always been a moderate drinker. I became suicidal ending up in psychiatric hospitals for 72 hour holds. Antidepressants were prescribed but nothing seemed to help. I was lost with no help to be found. This lasted for two and a half years. Then one afternoon I said to my husband "I need help." At 2:00 a.m. that night I was in the Psychiatric Crisis Unit being interviewed by an Intake Counselor. He asked is I thought I was an alcoholic and I said "no, I don't think so, I always quit when I get into trouble." He replied that I most certainly was and told me this based upon my history of hospitalizations, alcohol abuse, and an alcohol level upon intake to the hospital of .29. I asked what I should do. He said, "go to Alcoholics Anonymous."

I entered my first recovery meeting completely broken, humiliated and desperate. I reluctantly identified myself as "Rose" and listened intently. After the meeting I went up to the female secretary and asked if she would be my sponsor. She replied "yes" and thus began my recovery. I did everything that was suggested to me to do. That first night I went home and upon going to bed started drifting into that familiar dark depression. I called her and asked what I should do. She said to say the Third Step Prayer which I did turning my will and life over to God.

I felt a huge burden lift and I felt peace for the first time in years. That peace has continued since that day and a whole new life of love and service has emerged. I kept of a journal of my experiences, thoughts and feeling my first nine months of sobriety which became a book The **Gift of Sobriety: A Spiritual Transformation** published by Maple Leaf Publishing. The book has been very well received. I have a website at Rosesobriety.com which lists my blog (followed by 20,000+ people), reviews, radio interviews, a trailer and video. The book has been translated into French, Spanish, and Arabic. I have a film offer in English and French.

After one and a half years in recovery I began to feel a need to go deeper spiritually. I started attending the Center for Spiritual Living in Santa Rosa, California. I immediately related to the message and started taking a series of five classes. After studying for fifteen months I wrote a book of what I had learned: **My Spiritual Unfolding: Science of Mind**. This book has been picked up by NETFLIX for a series on TV.

I am now wanting to attend the Homes Institute to receive a Certificate in Spiritual Education. I am a life-long learner and want to continue to grow in my intellectual and experiential understanding of New Thought principles. This program seems to just be the right next step for me. I hope to continue writing about what I learn and be of service at the Center for Spiritual Living as I deepen my understanding of this philosophy.

I hope that I am accepted into the Certificate for Spiritual Education. Thank you.

Rose Bruce

I think that perhaps this pandemic is the earth's way of fighting back at humanity. We have destroyed our earth with pollution from cars and oil refineries. The ocean is full of plastics and global warming has cause the temperature of the earth to increase. Coral in the ocean are dying. Hurricanes, tornadoes and fires are more prevalent and bigger than ever before. It is predicted that the oceans will rise to the point that the islands and coastlines will disappear. The polar ice caps are melting. There are many endangered species that are disappearing as well.

Endangered Species Directory

Common name	Scientific name	Conservation status ↓
Amur Leopard	Panthera pardus orientalis	Critically Endangered
Black Rhino	Diceros bicornis	Critically Endangered
Bornean Orangutan	Pongo pygmaeus	Critically Endangered
Cross River Gorilla	Gorilla gorilla diehli	Critically Endangered
Eastern Lowland GorillaGorilla	beringei graueri	Critically Endangered
Hawksbill Turtle	Eretmochelys imbricate	Critically Endangered
Javan Rhino	Rhinoceros sondaicus	Critically Endangered
Orangutan	Pongo abelii, Pongo pygmaeus	Critically Endangered
Saola	Pseudoryx nghetinhensis	Critically Endangered
Sumatran Elephant	Elephas maximus sumatranus	Critically Endangered

Common name	Scientific name	Conservation status ↓
Sumatran Orangutan	Pongo abelii	Critically Endangered
Sumatran Rhino	Dicerorhinus sumatrensis	Critically Endangered
Sunda Tiger	Panthera tigris sondaica	Critically Endangered
Vaquita	Phocoena sinus	Critically Endangered
Western Lowland Gorilla	Gorilla gorilla Gorilla	Critically Endangered
Yangtze Finless Porpoise	Neophocaena asiaeorientalis ssp. Asiaeorientalis	Critically Endangered
African Wild Dog	Lycaon pictus	Endangered
Asian Elephant	Elephas maximus indicus	Endangered
Black-footed Ferret	Mustela nigripes	Endangered
Blue Whale	Balaenoptera musculus	Endangered
Bluefin Tuna	Thunnus Thynnus	Endangered
Bonobo	Pan paniscus	Endangered
Borneo Pygmy Elephant	Elephas maximus borneensis	Endangered
Chimpanzee	Pan troglodytes	Endangered
Fin Whale	Balaenoptera physalus	Endangered
Galápagos Penguin	Spheniscus mendiculus	Endangered
Ganges River Dolphin	Platanista gangetica gangetica	Endangered
Green Turtle	Chelonia mydas	Endangered
Hector's Dolphin	Cephalorhynchus hectori	Endangered
Humphead Wrasse	Cheilinus undulates	Endangered

Common name	Scientific name	Conservation status ↓
Indian Elephant	Elephas maximus indicus	Endangered
Indus River Dolphin	Platanista minor	Endangered
Irrawaddy Dolphin	Orcaella brevirostris	Endangered
Mountain Gorilla	Gorilla beringei beringei	Endangered
North Atlantic Right Whale	Eubalaena glacialis	Endangered
Red Panda	Ailurus fulgens	Endangered
Sea Lions	Zalophus wollebaeki	Endangered
Sea Turtle	Cheloniidae and Dermochelyidae families	Endangered
Sei Whale	Balaenoptera borealis	Endangered
Sri Lankan Elephant	Elephas maximus maximus	Endangered
Tiger	Panthera tigris	Endangered
Whale	Balaenoptera, Balaena, Eschrichtius, and Eubalaen	Endangered
Whale Shark	Rhincodon typus	Endangered
African Elephant	Loxodonta Africana	Vulnerable
Bigeye Tuna	Thunnus obesus	Vulnerable
Black Spider Monkey	Ateles paniscus	Vulnerable
Dugong	Dugong dugon	Vulnerable
Forest Elephant		Vulnerable
Giant Panda	Ailuropoda melanoleuca	Vulnerable
Giant Tortoise		Vulnerable

The virus is attacking all people around the world irrespective of boundaries. It is a global issue such as we have not faced since WW II. It is causing humanity to view itself as one group fighting this "enemy" together. The time for greed and nationalism is passing. It is estimated that the death rate from Covid-19 is 4%. If the world's population would shrink by 4% this would be a good thing for Mother Earth. We have been selfish and greedy for too long. Time for earth to rebalance and for humanity to learn to take care of all people not just the 1% that owns 99% of the world's wealth. It is a time to choose love instead of fear.

All over the world people are being ordered to "shelter in place" or stay at home. In the U.S. and other countries people can get fined or arrested if they do not have a valid reason for being out of doors. President Trump is thinking of having a quarantine in New York and New Jersey to contain the virus. New York has the most cases of any state.

The two-trillion-dollar-bill passed by Congress and the President yesterday is going to go to bail out the people, small and big businesses. Each adult who pays taxes and earns under $75,000 will get a check of $1200. Last week 3.5 million Americans filed for unemployment. It is now illegal to evict people for not paying their rent.

I am keeping sane by attending two recovery meetings today online at Zoom. It is so reassuring to see friend's faces and especially to see them in their homes.

Sunday, March 29, 2020

"GOOD COUNSEL- Today I give up the idea that I can be misled. With this freedom, I go within for guidance and listen to the great wisdom of Spirit within me."

I awoke in the night and decided to order a treadmill. The virus is spreading, "shelter in place" may last a month or two. We are not even allowed to walk around the neighborhood. There is no way I can go that long without working out. I have worked out nearly every day of my life. It will be hard to wait until next Thursday, April 2, 2020 when it is due to arrive. This gives me hope.

The Pope and the head of the World Health Organization are asking all countries to follow a ceasefire of all conflict. It is a time for peace, time to work for the common good of survival of the human race. Economies are collapsing temporarily but people are afraid about how they will support their families during this time. It is estimated that the unemployment rate will reach 20% during the peak of this crisis. It is predicted that the economy will bounce back in a few months when people can get back to work. That seems like a long time from now.

I have been feeling weak and achy so am staying in bed all day today which is highly unusual for me. Eric is up North taking care of him mom this weekend and I have no responsibilities I need to fulfill. Normally I would be going to the Center for Spiritual Living and taking Lee and Julie with me. Julie has the Covid-19 virus. I talked with her several times yesterday. Her boyfriend is taking care of her but there is not much he can do. Hospitals are not accepting any more patients now so people just have to wade it out as best they can. You can call your doctor and try to get antibiotics if necessary. She called her doctor and he has not returned her call in three days. Doctors and nurses are getting exhausted and sick. How long can this go on? Unfortunately for months.

The number of cases in the U.S. has reached 132,637 this morning with 2,351 deaths. Dr. Fauci, the head of the effort nationally, has predicted that as many as 200,000 people will dies in the U.S. I am going to start an Excel chart of cases and deaths each day for the world and the U.S. I can then create a chart to represent the steep curve that is happening. The goal of social isolation is to "flatten the curve" or spread out the number of cases over time so as to not overwhelm the hospitals. It is already too late for that in most parts of the U.S.

Everyone is making sacrifices by staying indoors and trying to help their neighbors and friends. It is a shift in consciousness away from self and to service. Of course, some people are stuck in fear. But I think most people are doing their best to stay in peace and service instead of fear. This is a wonderful thing.

The country is now looking at this outbreak as being in three phases. Phase 1 is spread of infections, which we are in now. Phase 2 is when the number of cases drops off for a period of two weeks and then social distancing can loosen up, people can go back to work and school. Phase 3 is lifting restrictions. The economic aid package to the nation has tripled the national debt. Although I did not live through World War II I heard about it from my parents and in movies. We are living through a similar time.

God bless us all.

I am finding myself feeling incredibly thankful for all of the goodness in my life: our home, landscaped yards, a hot tub, food to eat, heat, health, friends, a hot shower, shampoo, conditioner, perfume, a warm sweater... I suddenly realize how I've taken this all for granted and there is no assurance that it will continue to be so good. It probably will, of course. But right now, all of that feels so fragile.

I rested today and the aching has stopped. I feel healthy again, thank God. So many people are sick and dying. I do not want to watch any more news on TV about the coronavirus.

I think tomorrow I will start studying Science of Mind by Ernest Holmes. It is heavy reading and something I can sink my teeth into. I refuse to go under because of this virus. I've handled so many challenges in my life and this is just one more. I need to stay focused, disciplined, and smart.

I have not been in this house so many hours straight in a row since Leslie, my wife of twenty years, died. I have been keeping myself away from the house as much as possible to avoid the pain. Eric is gone now and that is part of the issue. I will feel better when he returns tomorrow. I just need to keep my head.

Friends on the Zoom calls who live alone are describing how difficult it is to be alone so long. I now understand what they are talking about. Right now, I am watching a series on TV that is free during this time. It is called The Affair and has many episodes. I am getting lost in this for a while but tomorrow I will be more disciplined. It is weird to have so many hours to fill and nowhere to go to fill them. Thank God I have this book to write!

Monday, March 30, 2020

"BODY — Today, I give up the idea that my body should be any different than what it is. I dedicate today to appreciating my body and noticing the endless number of ways in which it is a miracle."

I am on a news diet. I had gotten myself fixated on this pandemic and that is not healthy mentally. Let our elected officials deal with it. I need to deal with my mental health.

I went out into the yard and it is beautiful! I live on a third of an acre in Sonoma County, California: God's country. There are green rolling hills outside the large windows in the living room and dining room. I do not have blinds except to keep out the heat in the summer. Mostly I have the views to look at. To the West I can see the sunsets over the Pacific Ocean. I have white giant calla lily around my yard that are from three to five feet high. They bloom in the Spring and Fall. There is a vine with white flowers that I planted seven years ago that has now climbed up the two stories to the back deck and onto the canopy. It provides shade in the afternoon for the dining table there. It is so beautiful and I can see it from the dining room table where I study. The roses are starting to sprout new leaves to provide a supply of fresh roses for the dining room table. I have about twenty rose buses along the front curb. The long-stemmed red roses by the front porch are already blooming. The Gravenstein and Fuji apple trees and cherry tree are blossoming. I also have two ponds with lily pads and water lily plants in them. Recently we bought ferns to go around the ponds and last spring some bamboo shoots shot up thirty feet high around the ponds. We have a patio on the upstairs deck and downstairs deck with tables and chairs so we are ready to entertain at any time. I also love playing my 1939 restored Chickering Baby Grand piano. When this pandemic passes we will have a big BBQ and invite all of our friends.

Here are some pictures of our home. This is the view from the front living room window. Notice the beautiful roses curbside.

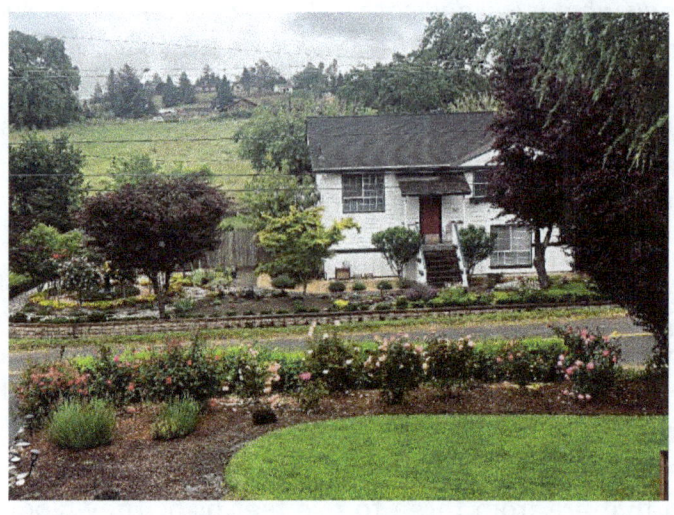

The front door steps and plants.

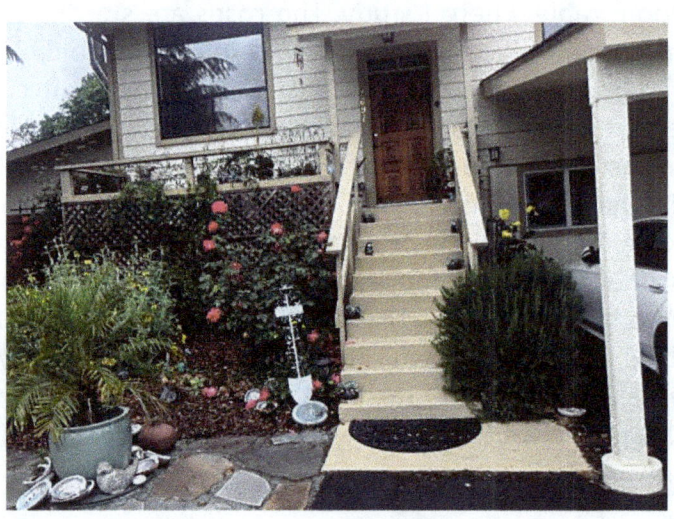

A peach tree in the backyard with calla lillys growing into it.

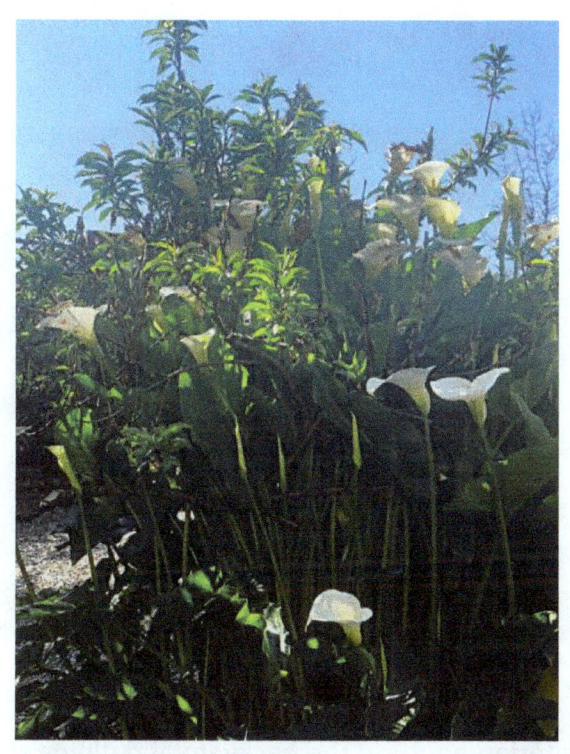

Gravenstein apple tree with calla lillys.

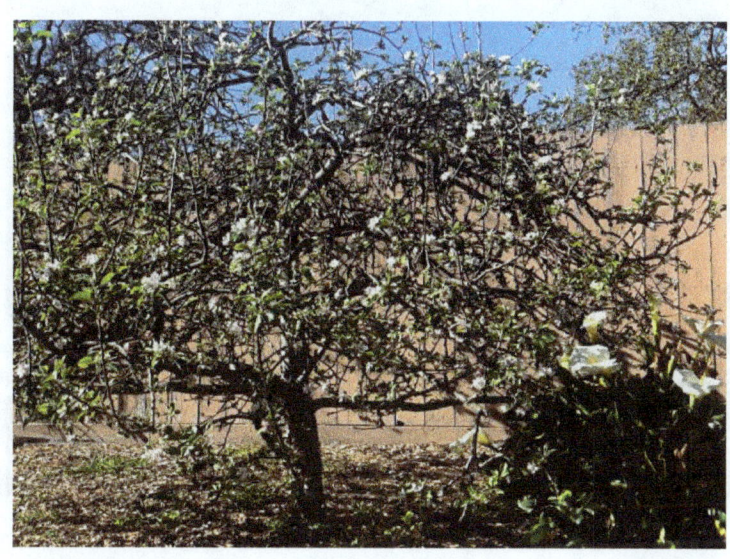

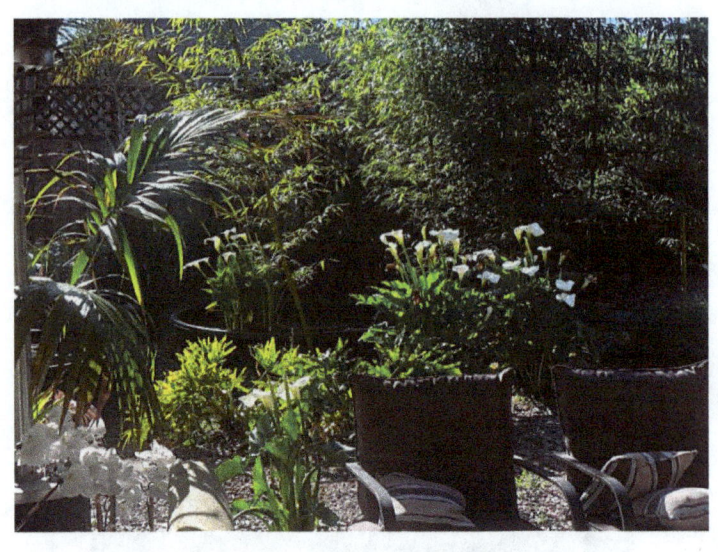

Meditation ponds in the backyard and dining room.

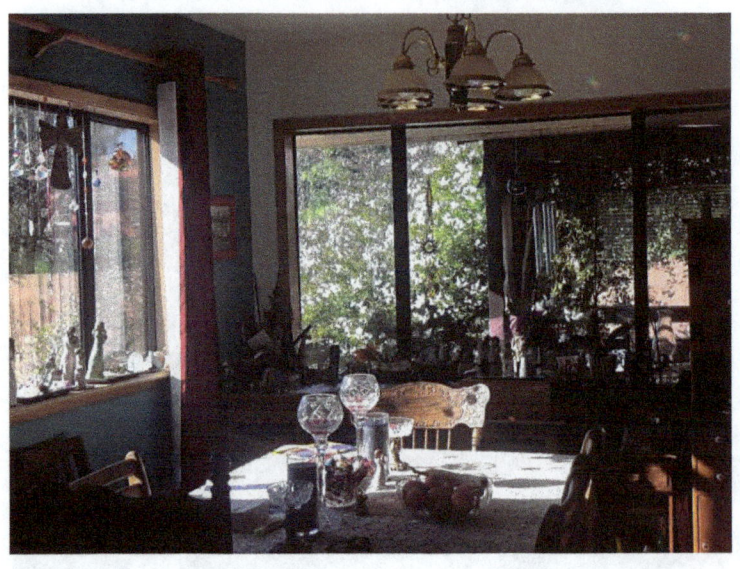

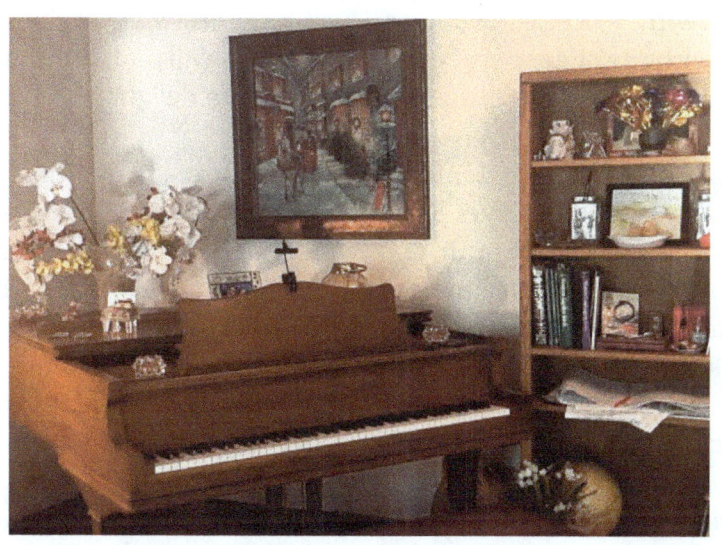

Restored 1935 Chickering Baby Grand piano.

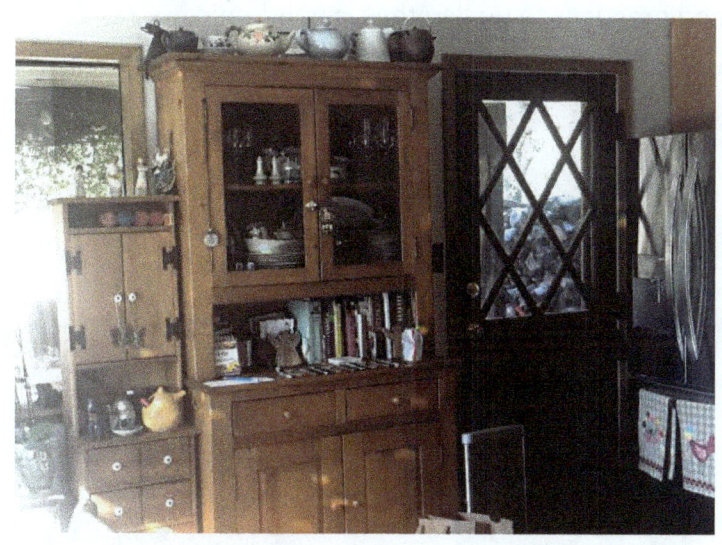

Amish hutch and spice rack in kitchen.

I pulled some frozen chicken out of the frig to fix tonight. Eric will return with groceries today so I will have fresh vegetables to fix along with the cheese stuffed pasta. I think I will pour alfredo sauce over the chicken and pasta for a special taste delight.

I am now going to continue reading spiritually uplifting books: Love Without End: Jesus Speaks by Glenda Green, Practicing the Presence by Joel Goldsmith, *Can We Talk God* by Ernest Holmes, Sermon *and the Mount* by Emmet Fox, and *Scientific Christian: Mental Practice* by Emma Curtis Hopkins. From these great resources. I have learned that "Thy Grace is my sufficiency" is a positive meditative phrase to turn to when I feel in lack or fear. I am returning to meditation and sacred books for inspiration and strength.

This afternoon at 2:00 p.m. I will have a facetime meeting with my sponsee Sandy. She is doing so well. She has just finished the twelve steps and is ready to start being a sponsor herself. Then at 6:30 p.m. I will log onto a Zoom recovery meeting where my sponsor will be attending. The sense of community is even stronger during these times. I am so blessed to be in recovery and have the tools and practices to deal with this pandemic.

Tuesday, March 31, 2020

"WEALTH – Today, I give up the idea that my wealth comes from anywhere other than the Radiant Presence of God within. I remain open and receptive to my source of supply. Spirit within is my wealth."

While the virus continues to spread and take its toll some positive things are happening. Yo-Yo Ma, a famous Cellist, started a website online called Songs of Comfort where he played a song for the world. Then Paul Simon added his song about America. And people all around the world are recording their songs of truth and meaning on the site. Elton John had an online concert that raised one million dollars to help with the pandemic. CEOs and Managers for department stores are forfeiting their salaries while they employees are furloughed. One NFL player donated half of his salary to the pandemic relief. Health care professionals are being so brave going to care for sick people without proper supplies, personal protective equipment (PPE), and overcrowded hospitals. Citizens are starting to applaud them at shift changes letting them know how much they are appreciated. Neighbors are scheduling times to go out on their balconies to play a song they all know and share. Neighbors are checking on each other, especially the elderly, to see if they need anything. Teachers are contacting students via email and holding classes via Zoom while parents are helping their children continue learning at home. People are volunteering to pass out boxes of food at the Food Banks while others are waiting in line for hours to receive the donation.

At home Eric and I are "nesting." We cleaned out a cupboard in the kitchen that contained old medicine and vitamins and moved the dishes around. That prompted a straightening of three other cabinets. He fertilized all of the rose bushes with rose bloom before the rain falls again tomorrow. He is straightening the garage which he has meant to get to for years. I am baking and cooking as I haven't done in years.

I could not find my mother's recipe for cherry oatmeal desert so call my sister Diane to get it from her. It was such fun talking with her. Her husband died suddenly a year and a half ago and we now talk every Sunday night. Today we just enjoyed sharing the recipe and talking about how we are coping.

Mom's Cherry Oatmeal Dessert

Topping: 1½ c flour, 1½ c oatmeal, 1 c brown sugar, ½ t soda, ½ t salt, 1 c melted butter, 1 c chopped walnuts. Combine and pour ¾ of mixture into a 8"X8"X2" pan.

Add 2 cans pie cherries mixed with 1t almond extract.

Top with remaining topping.

Bake @ 350 for 45 minutes.

Eric is getting text messages from High School friends he hasn't seen since the 30th High School Reunion this last October. Three have died from Covid-19 so far. He went to school in Sonoma, California just forty -five minutes from here so he is close. But we all get busy with our lives and drift apart. This pandemic is reminding us of how much we need each other.

While the world in facing an unprecedented crisis, we are reminded of what our values are and what is important in our lives: loved one, enough to eat, caring for others, remaining positive, keeping faith that this will pass and we will recover, most of us anyway. The human and economic toll is staggering yet we keep going in faith and trust.

Wednesday, April 1, 2020

"INSPIRED — Today, I give up the idea that I need to be inspired to express my greatness. I look within and find that the infinite Mind of God within me has never stopped providing me with inspiration, ideas, and newness. I consider myself to be highly blessed."

To me this time feels like a retreat. I have withdrawn from all outside activities and am focusing on my inner thoughts. I am also organizing the house as has not been done in years. It feels wonderful. It is a chance for Eric and I to make this our home together. He has lived here for about five years but became my husband only three years ago. For the first two years it was temporary and he brought his things down piecemeal. Today I took six large trash bags of clothes out of a closet upstairs, Leslie's clothes, my old professional clothes, and Leslie's mom's clothes. This will make more room for Eric to put hang up his t-shirts like he prefers to do. I think that's the last thing to do inside. We put some bulbs that had arrived in the mail into glass containers in the living room front window where the sun shines in. We are watching them shoot up each day. The bulbs are for Giant Globe flowers which will be four feet high with bright blue bulbs on top.

It feels really good to stop life for a while and go inward. I had developed a very busy lifestyle. Everyday had an outside activity. I usually began my day with prayer and meditation. Then I drove to Santa Rosa, a half hour away, and take an hour and a half walk around Spring Lake. It is a peaceful way to begin my day. Then lunch at Marvins, a local Mexican diner famous for its large portions and wonderful omeletes, where I know the waitresses and regulars. It feels like one large family. Afternoon and evening activities include seeing my sponsees, going to recovery meetings, regular household maintenance, answering emails, writing in my latest book, attending a class at the Center for Spiritual Living, doing homework, watching the PBS Newshour, and going to church.

Thursday afternoons we drive up the windy Highway 1 along the Pacific Coast up to Fort Bragg for dinner. It is three hours up and back each way and we love spending that time with each other away from cell phones and commitments. Eric and I go to couple's therapy once a week. We have found that with both of us being in sobriety and his mom having Alzheimers we are needing to learn how to handle new feelings. Eric is particularly troubled by his mom's illness. He spends at least two days a week up there plus arranging and taking her to all doctor's appointments here in Santa Rosa. I used to go with him but now feel better staying home focusing on my life. Then I have the reserves to take care of him emotionally when he returns burnt out and tired. I have a commitment at two recovery meetings a week. And I give rides to Lee and Julie to the Center for Spiritual Living on Sundays. I post something positive and thoughtful each week on my website at Rosesobriety.com. I have 20,000 readers following my blog and feel a sense of responsibility to them. It is a very full week. Recently I have been thinking about pulling back a bit. But in general, I like this pace in life – involved.

I like a quiet house while I am working. I do not like the TV on during the day. It is a time for me to think and reflect. I am an introvert and prefer my own company most of the time. At night we usually watch a movie or TV series like The Affair or The Crown. I hate sitcoms. They are an insult to my intelligence.

Now my days are totally different. I sleep in, as always, pray and meditate. But we are not allowed outside so I need to go in the back and front yards for my connection to nature. Fortunately, both are landscaped so I am surrounded by beauty. I have started drinking a cup of coffee in the morning which I had stopped for years. It tastes so good. But I need to be careful about consuming stimulants as I naturally have an abundance of energy. I oftentimes write in this book or study a spiritual book I am reading. I am cleaning, cooking and baking more. I feel very centered. I do not feel afraid unless I go to the grocery store or pharmacy and am reminded of the pandemic. Shelves are empty. People are standing three feet apart. There are very few shoppers. My treadmill comes tomorrow and I can't wait to hop on it.

I will probably go back to my workout routine I had while I was working which was doing the treadmill hill pattern each day for thirty intense minutes. It is a good workout. I walk around hills at Spring Lake so it will keep my legs in shape plus my cardio.

Mostly, I am feeling blessed. I am blessed to be healthy, have a home, to be financially secure, to have this book and the other two to deal with, spiritual books to read, recovery meetings to attend on Zoom. I am applying for the Certificate in Spiritual Education program at the Holmes Institute which should be very stimulating. I plan to begin this Fall 2020. Our home is so beautiful inside and out that I feel like I am living in a Better Homes and Garden life. It has taken twenty years to get it this way. I am aware of and thankful for this abundance every day. It is a rich, peaceful life.

I see other women in recovery at the Zoom meetings and they are having to live in their cars because they are homeless. Or they have children at home which is very demanding. Thank God that is not my lot. I like peace and quiet.

I can't wait until this is all over so we can have a big BBQ for our friends. Our home is well suited for outdoor entertaining and we are all missing each other. It WILL happen.

It is time to tune back into the news. The number of Covid-19 cases and deaths worldwide and in the U.S. has suddenly jumped. Is this because we have started testing? I have kept track of numbers since March 24, 2020, until today, or for the past two weeks. The charts of cases and deaths are below. There was a dramatic jump in both cases and deaths yesterday. I will continue to chart these changes.

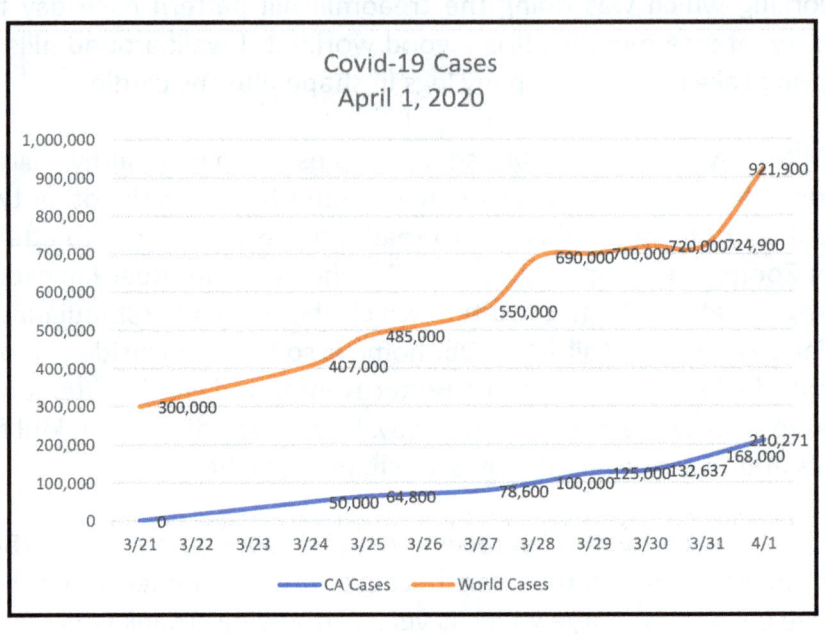

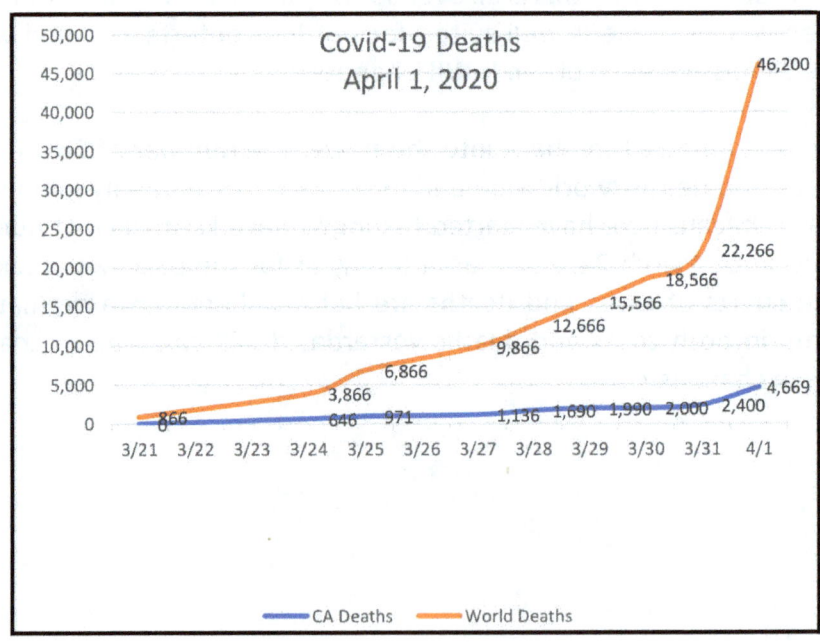

Hospitals are not having enough masks for healthcare professionals. People are being asked to sew their own masks. All N-95 masks are needed by the frontline workers. We are being told to donate them to hospitals rather than use them for personal care. Hospitals are calling upon construction workers and body shop workers to donate their face masks to the hospital.

The Wimbleton tennis playoffs in London were cancelled for the first time in their history. The U.S. census has been postponed as workers cannot go door to door to collect data.

People are finding creative ways to connect socially online. One DJ was spinning music for virtual dance parties and got 100,000 followers. One twelve year old girl's mom asked friend's parents to drive by during her birthday honking and yelling "happy birthday." David Hockney, a British artist on lockdown in France, is doing a series of artwork on Spring on his laptop and posting them. They are very popular and uplifting.

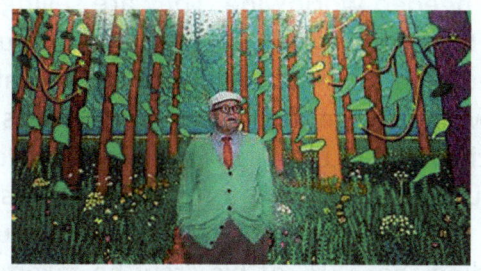

https://www.thetimes.co.uk/article/david-hockney-review-to-look-at-the-artists-new-spring-ipad-pictures-is-to-feel-the-spirit-lift-hqvgr503g

Friday, April 3, 2020

"ALIVE – Today, I give up those ideas that interfere with my ability to enjoy and express love. I am alive with divine energy, and with every breath I take, I see more clearly that I am alive in God."

Business have closed including restaurants, small businesses, bars, workout clubs, drive through restaurants, et cetera. Driving down the street I see dark, closed storefronts. When Eric was driving through Middletown on the way to see his mom Saturday, businesses were for sale. It is a small town and they cannot survive being closed a month or two.

Employees are being laid off in great numbers. In the U.S. last week 6.6 million people applied for unemployment insurance. This has doubled in the last week. Ten million people in the U.S. are out of work.

The Democratic Convention to select the candidate for the national presidential election in November was postponed a month. Ventilators are needed worldwide. They are selling for $35,000 to $50,000 each. President Trump is being asked to use his wartime authority to federalize companies to make ventilators. Blood donations are low and desperately needed. Labcorps and Quest are backlogged with Covid-19 tests causing some people to wait twelve days to get results. Children are not going back to school this year. The Captain of the USS Theodore Roosevelt sent out a letter a few days ago pleading that 90% of his crew be taken off of the ship because Covid-19 cases were starting to appear on ship and there was no way he could keep social distancing on the ship. This caused great alarm to families who heard about it on the news. Today that Captain Brett Crozier was fired for "overreacting" and "not being professional" or "going outside the chain of command."

Last Friday the Congress passed a bill and President Trump signed it giving 2.2 trillion in aid to Americans Federal Stimulus 2020. In California Governor Newsom is doing wonderful things to help citizens with unemployment and business shutdowns.

https://www.gov.ca.gov/california-takes-action-to-combat-Covid-19/

The State is providing $50 million in loan guarantees for small businesses who may not be eligible for federal relief. California is also allowing small businesses to defer payment on sales and use tax for up to $50,000 for up to 12 months. There is now $17.8 million in State initiatives to help workers impacted by Covid-19.

People are getting restless and frightened. They are wanting to escape. It is not surprising that the sale of alcohol in the U.S. went up 55% last week. I understand. I used alcohol for thirty-five years, from thirty to sixty-five. It was my "go-to" to celebrate, relax, socialize, unwind, or generally not face what I was dealing with for a while. I had two to three glasses of wine every night. My drinking got worse toward the end of my career when I was feeling increased pressure and dissatisfaction. Then my life partner and wife of twenty years, Leslie, died of cancer and I was devastated. I was also retired. Life held no meaning for me and I abused alcohol to "cope." It did not work. I got worse, ended up with suicide attempts and hospitalizations, and finally referral to Alcoholics Anonymous. I still did not think I was an alcoholic. I could not imagine getting through life without it.

There is a brief survey, Twenty Questions, that I took upon beginning recovery. It is The Johns Hopkins Twenty Questions: Are You An Alcoholic? It was developed in the 1930s by Dr. Robert Seliger, who at that time was a faculty member in the Department of Psychiatry at the Johns Hopkins Hospital. It was intended for use as a self-questionnaire to determine the extent of one's use of alcohol.

TWENTY QUESTIONS

1. Have you lost time from work because of your drinking?
2. Is drinking making your home life unhappy?
3. Do you drink because you are shy with other people?
4. Is drinking affecting your reputation? 5. Have you ever felt remorse after drinking?
6. Have you gotten into financial difficulties because of drinking?
7. Do you turn to lower companions or environment when drinking?
8. Does your drinking make you careless of your family's welfare?
9. Has your ambition decreased since drinking?
10. Do you crave a drink at a definite time of day?
11. Do you want a drink the next morning?
12. Does drinking cause you to have difficulty sleeping?
13. Has your efficiency decreased since drinking?
14. Is drinking jeopardizing your job or business?
15. Do you drink to escape from worries or trouble?
16. Do you drink alone?
17. Have you ever had a complete loss of memory as a result of drinking?
18. Has your physician ever treated you for drinking?
19. Do you drink to build up your self-confidence?
20. Have you ever been to a hospital or institution because of drinking?

If you answer YES to any one of the questions, there is a definite warning that you may be an alcoholic.

If you answer YES to any two, the chances are that you are an alcoholic.

If you answer YES to three or more, you are definitely an alcoholic.

When I took it, I answered YES to 17 questions out of 20. Yet I did not want to admit to myself I was an alcoholic. I suspected it in the back of my mind. But I could not face that reality until it was shoved in my face.

Such is the denial and dependence in alcoholism and drug addiction. It can only be understood by another alcoholic. That is why getting into recovery and talking to other people who understand the disease is so helpful. It is a disease. There are genetic predispositions and it is progressive leading to insanity or death if untreated. The body of the alcoholic does not process alcohol the way a "normal" person does. In the alcoholic there is an allergy to alcohol that creates a craving in the body that is insatiable. It is very dangerous and little understood by the general public.

When I got into recovery, about seven months in, I realized the person I had hurt the most by my drinking was me. I had stopped growing in my ability to cope and had stymied my creativity. When I got sober, that all changed. I kept a journal of my recovery for the first nine months. It turned in to a book *The Gift of Sobriety: A Spiritual Transformation* available from Amazon, Barnes and Noble, by publisher Maple Leaf Publishing or from my website Rosesobriety.com. It has been translated into French, Spanish, and Arabic. It has gotten favorable reviews and is reaching an enthusiastic audience. A week ago, I was contacted by Westwood books to be on TV doing an interview about my book *The Gift of Sobriety: A Spiritual Transformation* and recovery. I am happy to do this. Especially at this time there is a great need.

I am retreating into my backyard for escape. The treadmill arrived yesterday and Eric set it up on the downstairs patio under the canopy. It looks out on the ponds, blossoming fruit trees, calla lillys, ferns and giant bamboo. I can hear the water running in the ponds as I work-out. I slept so much better last night having worked out my usual half hour at three miles per hour. I could feel it in my butt, thighs, and upper arms this morning. I just finished working out for today. It gives me energy and helps me to feel calm.

I noticed when I was checking out at Target that every other shopped had liquor in their basket, usually hard liquor. I understand their intent but it won't work to make the situation better. It only makes things worse.

In California the cannabis average order sales have increased 38% since March 16th due to the coronavirus. First-time deliveries were up 51% and the number of people signing up on Eaze website was up 105%.

The need for Personal Protective Equipment or PPE has increased dramatically. These are the N-95 masks, plastic gowns and gloves that are worn by front-line hospital doctors and nurses. Mayor Cuomo of New York, the epicenter of cases in the U.S., has asked private hospitals to give their PPEs to the public hospitals. States are out-bidding each other for this equipment. The federal stockpile is being "held back" for "just a back-up" according to President Trump and his son-in-law Jarad Kushner. This is making Governors and the American people very angry. Over half of Americans believe President Trump is doing a "poor" job of handling the pandemic. He has consistently given inaccurate information and misled the American people about the severity of the crisis. He was slow to respond with needed production of PPEs and ventilators. 3M has now been called upon by the Federal Protection Act to make face masks. And GM is making ventilators. Ventilators for New York are being bought from China because there is a shortage in the U.S.

Hospitals are starting to use plastic coats and garbage bags for PPEs. Citizens are making home-made face masks out of material and donating them to the hospitals as they are running out. Videos and guidelines for making masks are now online

https://www.cnn.com/2020/04/04/health/how-to-make-your-own-mask-wellness-trnd/index.html

Today President Trump ordered all Americans to wear face masks when they go out. These are regular face masks not the N-95 that are needed at the hospitals. Now 96% of Americans are honoring the "stay at home" order for the benefit of public health.

Dr. Andrew Fauci is the "face" on TV of Covid-19 information for the federal government. He has been a federal public health advisor since the 1980s when there was the AIDS epidemic. He is calm, factual and comforting. People are putting his face on mugs and t-shirts. He is the voice of reason. He is also receiving death threats because of the facts that he is presenting. Dr. Sanjay Gupta is also helping educate Americans with his podcasts Fact vs. Fiction on the coronavirus on CNN
https://www.cnn.com/2020/04/04/health/how-to-make-your-own-mask-wellness-trnd/index.html
The lack of ventilators is causing health professionals in the U.S. to prioritize who should get them. The virus are attacks the respiratory system causing people to have shortness of breath and trouble breathing. At some point the patient is either being put on a ventilator or left to die. Families are not being allowed into hospitals to comfort their dying members. Children and old people are dying alone. There was an article today in the New England Journal of Medicine by Dr. Robert Truog suggesting a "point system" to prioritize patients
https://www.nejm.org/doi/full/10.1056/NEJMp2005689

"The Centers for Disease Control and Prevention estimates that 2.4 million to 21 million Americans will require hospitalization during the pandemic, and experience in Italy has been that about 10 to 25% of hospitalized patients will require ventilation, in some cases for several weeks. On the basis of these estimates, the number of patients needing ventilation could range between 1.4 and 31 patients per ventilator. Whether it will be necessary to ration ventilators will depend on the pace of the pandemic and how many patients need ventilation at the same time, but many analyses warn that the risk is high." The "point system" would give elder Americans and those with preexisting conditions such as COPD a lower score."
The number of cases in the world and U.S. continues to rise. As of April 4 ,2020 there are 1,187,798 cases worldwide with 64,083 deaths. In the U.S. there are 301,902cases with 8,175 deaths, three times the number of deaths as after 911. New York has 113,000 cases with 3,500 deaths. The next two weeks are expected to be worse

Palm Sunday, April 5, 2020

"DIVINITY — Today, I give up the idea of Divinity as something far off and distant. I reaffirm that my mind is a center of divine activity within the mind of God, and I focus on the main ways I can express that through my actions, intentions, and words."

It is Palm Sunday and the churches are closed worldwide.

The most helpless in society are the poor and homeless. The Federal Stimulus Bill 2020 will help the poor in the U.S. But what about the homeless? In California Governor Newsom has taken measures to remove infected homeless people off of the streets and into housing. Currently there are 6,867 rooms in hotels and motels being rented by the State for homeless individuals with the virus. In Phase One there will be 15,000 beds. FEMA is paying 75% of the reimbursement for rooms for exposed homeless people.

Chef Jose Andreas, the founder of the World Central Kitchen, *https://wck.org* is feeding these homeless and others in need of a hot meal. He is a world-renowned chef who has in the past years gone into emergency situations to provide food. The World Central Kitchen has served 750,000 meals to vulnerable communities facing severe food insecurity such as in Puerto Rico after the hurricane two years ago. His organization is providing Covid-19 relief to New York City; Los Angeles; Washington DC; Little Rock, Arkansas; Oakland, California; New Orleans; St. John (USVI), Fairfax, Virginia; Boston and Madrid, Spain. He works with local authorities and volunteers to put hot meals into the hands of people who need it most.

Every adult in the U.S. who pays taxes and earns less than $75,000 per year will be getting a check for $1,200 within the next two weeks with $600 for each child in the household. This is part of the Federal Stimulus Bill 2020. Couples who earn less than $150,000 per year will get $2,400. This is to cover the cost of rent, food and medications.

There are federal guidelines prohibiting any landlord from evicting someone during this time. Water cannot be shut off in homes and businesses in California.

Foodbanks throughout the U.S. are handing out free food as never before *https://www.feedingamerica.org/find-your-local-foodbank* . The need is increasing every day. People are being turned away after the fool runs out.

Donations for all of these activities can be given online. Individuals and organizations are donating money. CNN has a site to donate at *https://www.cnn.com/impact*. The Bill and Melinda Gates Foundation has given over 100 million to help contain the outbreak of the coronavirus. NBA players are donating money to cover salaries of hourly workers impacted by ending the season early. The Late Show with Steven Colbert is accepting donations.

The earth is benefitting from the Covid-19 crisis. Entire large cities such as Wuhan, New York City, Paris, Moscow and Los Angeles are shut down. There are very few cars and factories are shut down so there is very little pollution going into the air. It will probably not have any long-term effect but in the short term the earth gets a break from our daily emissions insult.

Hearts everywhere are opening to help others. Neighbors are checking on each other and especially the elderly during this time. They are shopping for people who cannot go out. We are coming together as we only do in time of crisis such as a World War or this pandemic. Can we sustain this level of care? I hope so.

The past two days it has been raining. It feels to me like the heavens are crying for the dying. It is also washing away the virus. The next two weeks are forecast to be the worst for Covid-19 in the U.S. We are reaching the apex of the curve of infections and deaths. God help us all!

Cases	worldwide 1,272,115	U.S. 337,072
Deaths	worldwide 69,374	U.S. 9,619
Percent Deaths	worldwide 5.4%	U.S. 2.9%

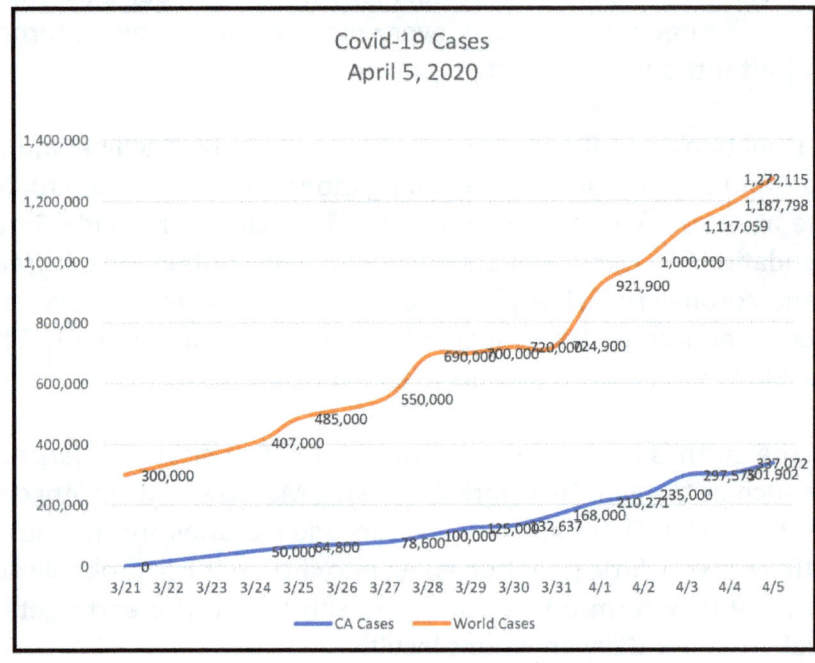

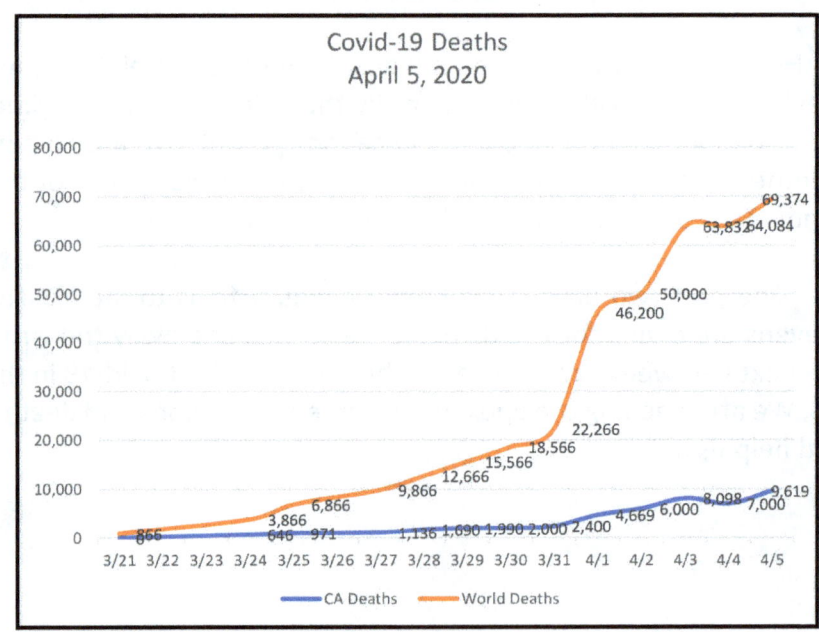

Monday, April 6, 2020

"LIVING PRESENCE — Today, I give up the idea that I am separate from God, and I embrace wholeheartedly the idea that my very nature is God's nature expressing as love, kindness, and vibrancy. I turn to the Presence within for guidance and inspiration.

The surgeon general of the U.S. has said that this next week will be "our Pearl Harbor moment" referring to the Japanese attack on Pearl Harbor that brought the U.S. into WW II. The number of cases and deaths are projected to rise dramatically. Americans are drawing together as never before since WW II to help us get through this with as little destruction as possible. There is an attitude of self-sacrifice for the common good. The newscasters on 60 Minutes last night said people from now on will refer to their lives as pre-Covid-19 and post-Covid-19. It is a defining moment in history. They took a moment of silence to recognize the collective grief that so many families are feeling now. Over 9,000 Americans have died in the last two weeks from Covid-19. That is incomprehensible. On the AMC Our Country concert on TV last night, in place of the scheduled American Music Awards which have been postponed until September 16, 2020, they used the phrase "we're all in this together." This sense of shared responsibility and caring is a gift of the virus. How sad that it took this to wake us up.

My daily routine has changed greatly over the course of the "stay-at-home" order. I start the day with prayer and meditation to discern how I might be of service today followed by a cup of coffee and a protein bar. I then write in this book notes from the night before. At 11:45 a.m. I tune into CNN to catch the latest national news. At noon I switch to KTVU Channel 2 for California news. Then I treadmill for a half hour, shower, and get back to work. I have a diet coke and check emails. There are about 20-30 each day with offers related to the crisis like selling face masks, buying life insurance and having daily news updates. At 3:00 p.m. I watch the *PBS Newshour* usually followed by the Steven Colbert Late Night Show from the night before for a funny take on the news to lift up my spirits.

Sundays I watch John Oliver's Last Week Tonight for another funny news source. In general, I am watching news much more than usual to have accurate information to report here. I watch in a detached manner as a Social Science researcher which is my professional training and experience for thirty years. I used to write research reports all year long as part of my normal workload. It is easy for me to do it now. I look for themes and facts. After I have written them down in here, I am able to forget them. It is not scarring my consciousness as it is for many people. It can be very damaging to watch too much news.

Today California is preparing for the next week of potential crisis. Governor Newsom has added 50,000 beds to the 75,000 hospital beds in 416 hospitals in the state. Sports arenas like the Sacramento Kings Basketball Stadium are being converted into alternative care sites. The most severe cases will remain at the hospitals where they have the staff to take care of them. Retired doctors and nurses are volunteering to help at these sites. California is sending 500 ventilators to the federal stockpile to be used by other states like New York or Michigan. Governor Newsom started preparing for this pandemic at the end of January this year when people from China on a cruise ship were detained for two weeks in quarantine. Unlike President Trump, he started early, much to our benefit in the state.

The Inspector General of the Federal Department of Health and Human Services released a report today on the preparedness of U.S. hospitals to handle the Covid-19 crisis. The 300 hospitals reporting cited "widespread" and "severe shortages of medical equipment". President Trump is getting increasing criticism for his poor handling of the national response. He failed to act in February while other Governors were reacting. He responded slowly and with inconsistent information. In early March President Trump called the corid-19 pandemic a "hoax" promulgated by the Democrats against him to keep him from getting reelected in November. He has routed ventilators from China to private companies for competitive bidding among state governors so states are now going directly to China themselves to procure this much needed equipment.

He has urged citizens to "go to work, even if you are sick, to keep the economy going." President Trump seems to make every comment about the virus to be about himself rather than the issues. He criticizes governors who do not "appreciate" the federal response and told Vice President Pence to "not call them back." President Trump last Friday suggested that Covid-19 victims take an anti-malaria drug hydroxychloroquine to combat the symptoms even though "there is no strong medical evidence that this is helpful." He prevented Dr. Fauci from answering questions about the drug during the press conference. Doctors are now hoarding the drug and people with lupus and rheumatoid arthritis who need the drug regularly and are now not able to get it so they are in pain. Some people have died from the drug. The American people (48%) are giving President Trump a "very bad" rating for his on handling of the pandemic.

Prime Minister Johnson of Great Britain is in critical condition in the hospital with Covid-19. He was seen shaking hands of people in the streets a week ago. He has signed his power to run the government over to Dominic Raab, the second in command. CNN's Chris Cuomo, the younger brother of Governor Andrew Cuomo is infected with coronavirus. [New York's Mayor is Bill de Blasio]

Today in the U.S. there are 367,507 cases for Covid-19 with 10,908 deaths. Just two weeks ago there were only three cases in the U.S.

Tuesday, April 7, 2020

"EMBODIMENT OF THE CHRIST – Today I give up the idea that the Christ is a particular person and realize that Christ is every person. I dedicate myself to seeing and loving Christ within everyone and everything."

I have spent the day rejuvenating myself. I have rested, read, written in this book, baked, cooked and played the piano. I am memorizing the piano piece Christofori's Dream by David Lanz. It is a beautiful and inspiring piece. I want to be able to sit down anywhere anytime and share its beauty with others.

It is important for me to take time to go within and recharge. I think this is true for everyone. But it is especially true for the introvert, like myself. I get rechanged by paying attention to my thoughts and reading inspiration material. Today it was Love Without End: Jesus Speaks by Glenda Green. This is a source of continual amazement to me. I am reading about the Sacred Heart.

> In the depths of your being is your own sacred center. It is the still, quiet chamber deep within where you are one with the Father...The very act of being there is the essence of prayer...

> The Sacred Heart has an exact location in the body which can very slightly in every person, but it is approximately the same. It is located in the space between the spine and the physical heart, anywhere from an inch above the physical heart to three inches below it...

> As you enter, you must release your attention into silence, letting it fall until it comes to rest. This is the way of quiet contemplation in which you may behold the oneness of all that is. This is your sacred place, for it is the pivotal link between the body and soul, the physical and the immortal, between yourself and God...

Inside the sacred silence you may experience bliss and quietness, and receive a healing, or nurturing...There are seven dimensions of intelligence which resonate outwardly from the center of your heart: unity, love, life, respect, honesty, justice, and kindness... You strengthen the heart through appreciation, acceptance and forgiveness.

It is so important that you respect your individuality and self-awareness that you possess. From that self-awareness you derive your capacity for thought and imagination. Contained within it is your right to be an additional source of infinity and creation. (pp. 163-164.)

Wednesday, April 8, 2020

"KINDNESS – Today I give up the idea that there is any other way for me to express myself than with my natural-born kindness. The Mind of God within me causes me to act with kindness."

Newscasters are starting to describe this Covid-19 reality as "the new norm." The world is changed forever by a "foreign invader." "We are at war" they cry. In Wuhan, China, where the virus started in December 2019, they lifted the "shelter at home" order today after eleven weeks, 76 days since January 21st. Citizens are still encouraged to stay at home if possible. Many are leaving the area to go home after travelling for Chinese New Year at the beginning of the outbreak. I think I will go crazy if I have to stay home for eleven weeks! Bill Gates, co-founder of Microsoft and philanthropist, said he thought we would be in this state of alert until we get a vaccine which could take from one to one and a half years. Yikes! On the other hand, yesterday Cuomo of New York said they may have reached their apex of cases which means things would go down from here. The number of deaths in New York rose to a record high in one day of 179.

I woke up this morning to the sound of the bi-weekly lawn maintenance crew working in my yard. How comforting to hear a "normal" sound. Time to get back to self-discipline. With the lack of external structure, I need to rely on internal structure to shape my days. I will go treadmill soon. Wednesday is laundry day so I will throw in a load of clothes on the way to workout. I will then practice the piano. I've nearly got the piece memorized. I will keep writing in this book which is like one long research report.

The fashion industry is citing severe drops in sales for clothes and furs. The stock market is, of course, still in trouble. The latest Dow was 22,818 points which is basically in the middle between the high and lows this year. Secretary of State Minuchin, the economic advisor to the President, is suggesting we need another $250 billion bailout for small businesses which impacts 90% of the U.S.

Although President Trump continues to insist there is "no problem" with the process for small businesses to apply for loans, business owners report that the process is "plagued by technical failure and confusion." There are reports of the funds going to companies listed on the Stock Exchange rather than the small businesses that it was intended to serve. Some of these large businesses are giving the money back to the federal government. Individuals applying for unemployment are reporting having to call the state hotline fifty times a day without success to complete their application. The federal infrastructure was not prepared for a pandemic.

Bernie Sanders dropped out of the Democratic Primaries yesterday. Former Vice-President Joe Biden is now the likely candidate to challenge President Trump in November. The influence of Bernie Sander's liberal agenda will be felt in the Democratic Party. Ideas like health care for all, free college tuition and addressing the global warming will likely be added to the Democratic Party ideology in November. With rallies cancelled, the candidates are having to rely on televised interviews to get their message out. President Trump is using his daily Covid-19 address to the nation as a political platform to get reelected. This is not appropriate and he is getting much public criticism for doing it.

The advertisements on TV reflect the Covid-19 issues already. They are aimed at selling items needed during this time such as delivery pizza or shoes needed by frontline responders. U.S. Olympic competitors are sharing positive statements of hope for when they will compete in Tokyo next year, one year later than scheduled. Twitter continues to have misinformation despite a promise it would stop doing so. Estimates are that 59% of the false statements are still being run. Facebook and YouTube are doing better with 24% and 27% respectively false information ads being continued.

Today's figures: worldwide 1,500,830 cases with 87,706 deaths or 5.8%. In the U.S. there are 423,135 cases with 14,390 deaths or 3.4%. I would say the earth is doing a pretty good job at reducing the world population. The earth IS alive, like any organism, and I believe it will protect itself from us humans.

I ran this theory by my friends and am surprised by how many say they have thought it but haven't dare mentioned it. John Prine, a famous Country Singer, died yesterday from the Covid-19 virus. He was 70 years old. His songs include Angel from Montgomery. The virus can be spread by individuals who do not show symptoms for a week. Flags are at half-mast throughout the country in honor of those who have died from the virus.

I am finding the Sacred Heart meditation to be very relaxing and rejuvenating. It gives me peace to focus on that instead of the negative stream of news blasting 24-7. This is a trying time and people are talking more and more about a spiritual response to cope. This is new in the popular news media. The world IS changing in a positive way now.

Thursday, April 9, 2020

"ETERNAL — Today, I give up the idea of beginnings and endings, and I notice how everything and everyone extends in every direction of time. I see how utterly beautiful life is.

I am tired of the pandemic defining my reality. I am stuck at home but I have freedom in my thoughts and actions. I shared the draft of this book with a colleague from Sonoma State University and he commented on how deeply personal it was. Yes, that is how I write now. My readers have come to expect it from me. One of the reason's I left academia was because I was so tired of just relying on the mind and ignoring the heart.

I think I will start the day with a treadmill workout followed by a hot shower...I started reading a fascinating book recommended by my colleague: Testimony of Light by Helen Greaves. It was communicated by telepathy from a nun who died and then communicated with her Sister what she was experiencing. It is a perfect read for these days...keeping life on this earth in perspective.

Ten percent of the U.S. workforce is now unemployed. Citizens cannot pay their rent. There is a moratorium on evictions for missed rent or mortgages payments. People are wondering if they can buy food and how they will ever recover from this setback. Property taxes are due April 15th and many people cannot pay them. The Federal Reserve has made available $2.2 trillion in loans available for small businesses. This is unprecedented and the worse since the great depression. Ninety seven percent of Americans are staying home to help prevent the spread of Covid-19. This is becoming the new norm.

In the U.S. there are 462,000 cases with 16,500 deaths. It is reported that if one is infected, for the first week there are no visible symptoms. Then symptoms appear for a week. For many people they need to go to the hospital at this time period. For others they die one week later. It is a grim progression.

Good Friday, April 10, 2020

"AWARENESS — Today, I give up the idea that my mind is separate from the all-knowing Mind of God. I practice noticing the power, truth, and beauty in my thought. I dedicate my awareness of the recognition of God's power and presence."

There is a sense of expansiveness to my day now that I have never experienced before except for briefly while on vacations. There are no "required" activities that I must perform. Even in retirement I have structured my life so as to have external demands and commitments each day. Now there are endless hours of leisurely contemplation and reflection. I reflect on the new book I am reading. I reflect on the pandemic. But mostly there is a feeling of leisure such as I've never known before. How luxurious life seems. Such a gift. Perhaps that is part of what this pandemic can teach us: to slow down and enjoy life. I notice the lizards sunning themselves on the fence outside. I listen to the water flowing in the ponds by the downstairs patio. I see the new leaves on the apple tree when I work out. I am NOTICING life instead of racing through it. What a gift!

I just read a statement in Testimony of Light that seemed like it could have been taken from Ernest Holmes' writing.

> "In the human mind, a negative thought can creep in and insinuate itself between all one's good intentions, lying apparently dormant. Then it becomes a nucleus attracting to itself thought of similar content until it takes on a semblance of force through emotion; later the results, physical, material or spiritual are manifested." (p. 71.)

This reminds me to what I wrote at the end of my last book *My Spiritual Unfolding: Science of Mind* on Mind Treatment.

What is Treatment?

The world's great religions agree that there is one creative intelligence that underlies all reality. It is called many different names: God, Allah, Yahweh, Jehovah, First Cause, Chi, Qi, Adonai, Hashem, Krishna, Buddha nature, Tao, the I AM. God is ever present, all knowing, and all powerful. It is power, beauty, light, love, benevolence, kindness, forgiveness, peace, and serenity. It is ever drawing us closer to Itself.

Ernest Holmes distilled this understanding into the Science of Mind philosophy. He states that in the macrocosm the Word, or First Cause, is the origin of all that has ever existed or will ever exist. It is eternal. Thought preceeds manifestation. In the microcosm humans create their life experiences by their thoughts conscious and unconscious. Most of our deepest thoughts about ourselves come from our family and society and are unconscious. We accept on some level that we are not good enough; that we are inferior because of the color of our skin, our gender, our sexual orientation, our disabilities…that we are not worthy. These thought forms are creating our existence oftentimes beyond our awareness. Therefore, it is essential that we bring to consciousness our assumptions about life and ourselves.

Ernest Holmes and others in the New Thought movement teach that we can heal ourselves and others through the use of Affirmative Prayer called Spiritual Mind Treatment. In this process the Practitioner claims for themselves and the other the reality of their Divine Existence devoid of illness of lack of any kind.

Emmet Fox in his book The *Sermon on the Mount* states that Jesus taught spiritually or metaphysically. Fox states that serenity is "tranquility of the soul." "To pray scientifically means to affirm that God is helping us, that temptation has no power against us, and to constantly claim that our own real nature is spiritual and perfect (p. 55). "

In The Lord's Prayer Jesus teaches us to accept each day our daily bread. We are to expect that God will provide us fully with everything we need. "Bread does not merely mean food but all that that we require for a healthy, happy, free, and harmonious life. This includes food, clothing, shelter, means to travel, books, and so on; above all, we require freedom" (Fox, p. 162). We are free to choose to accept the Divine Goodness or rely on our own self for supply.

Surrender is required in order to experience God's perfect Grace. Most us of surrender a little bit at a time. We may pray in the morning, meditate for a half hour, go to yoga class, and give thanks in the evening. We may experience peace and serenity at these times. Then we go back to our normal experiences of reality, strife, and anxiety. Emerson states "our faith comes in glimpses while our vices are perpetual." We are instructed by Jesus to" pray without ceasing." We are to live in the Presence of God every moment of our lives.

For others surrender is complete and sudden. This opening is prompted by a feeling of desperation and the awareness that all that has had meaning in one's life before makes no sense, has led to failure, lack, and often suicidal ideation. This awareness makes the person open to receive God's Grace and learn a new way of life. It is a gift of desperation that creates a willingness to release our hold on our old life and let God take over. There is a shattering of the illusion of separateness and a restoration of the soul to its wholeness.

What are we to do when we experience lack? Joel Goldsmith in his book Practicing the Presence writes "The spiritual life reveals clearly that God's grace is our sufficiency in all things. We do not need anything in this world except His grace" (p. 83). When we experience lack, we are to declare unreservedly that "Thy Grace is my sufficiency." Jesus teaches us "Seek ye first the kingdom of God and all else will be given unto you."
In Love Without End: Jesus Speaks by Glenda Green we read that Jesus told her that,

at the center of your soul is the Sacred Heart. This is the point at which you are one with God. The heart sees infinity within and without...It can ascertain the origin of conditions and change them. The heart is your higher intelligence... Your mind is merely a servant and it behaves well if it is given positive impulses; it behaves very poorly if it is given negative impulses...It is from this power, within the center of your being that the entire script of your life is written. Live in your heart to either fulfill the script of your life or to rewrite it... The answers to healing your life will be found in the inner strength of your heart...Strengthen all of your positive emotions through daily gratitude and admirations. Disempower your negative emotions daily through forgiveness. (pp. 50-51).

Ernest Holmes in Can We Talk To God? writes "The secret of spiritual power is a consciousness of one's union with the whole and the availability of good" (p. 58). I think that in Spiritual Mind Treatment the power comes from dropping into our Sacred Heart and realizing our Divinity and the Divinity of those we treat. We then affirm the reality of the Goodness that comes from that Divine Inheritance. We place the mind in its proper place as a servant to our positive thoughts thereby stimulating the Law of Life to create that which we know to be true.

Ads on TV are increasingly being about support and thanks for the people who are working to get us all though this pandemic: hospital staff, grocery store workers, FedEx drivers and food delivery people. Two days ago, there was a primary election in Wisconsin. They tried to postpone it but the Supreme Court in the state denied the proposal. Voters were forced to risk their lives to cast their votes. It is considered a disgrace.

The Pope gave a talk from closed-circuit TV for Good Friday. Crude oil prices have dropped 50% since the pandemic. Saudi Arabia and others are stopping production of oil by 10% per day in hopes of boosting the prices. David Brooks on PBS Newshour reported a poll he took of New York Times readers of mental health in reaction to the pandemic. Young people are feeling hopeless and are crying all day, senior citizens feel a sense of isolation with "shelter in place" orders, and those with mental health problems reports exacerbation of symptoms. Response ratings for state Governors are high while ratings of President Trump's response are low. President Trump is requiring "North Korean loyalty" of those around him firing anyone who does not support him 100%. Saudi Arabia and Yemen have declared a cease fire because of the pandemic.

Cases continue to rise. There are 1,650,210 cases worldwide with 100,376 deaths. In the U.S. there are 473,093 cases with 17,836 deaths.

Saturday, April 11, 2011

"I let go and see the evidence of Love in action all around me. The love of the Divine inspires me to express my love for self, others, and for life itself."

I just came from a recovery meeting online. It is so reassuring to see my "family" of friends again.

Cases continue to rise worldwide and nationally. Worldwide there are 1,754,457 cases with 107,520 deaths, 6.1%. In the U.S. there are 514,4153 cases with 19,882 deaths, 3.9%. Below are the charts that represent the continuing trend upwards. The number of deaths is rising sharply as people who were sick die from the Covid-19 virus. The increase in deaths is staggering and can only be grasped by looking at the visual in the chart below or hearing the grief in the voices of family members on the news. There is one promising treatment for the disease: taking antibodies in the blood of someone who has recovered and injecting it into a sick person. One person in Washington treated this way reversed from positive to negative in ONE DAY! Doctors are also doing clinical trials on the hydroxychloroquine that President Trump is recommended to see how effective it MIGHT be. No results as of yet.

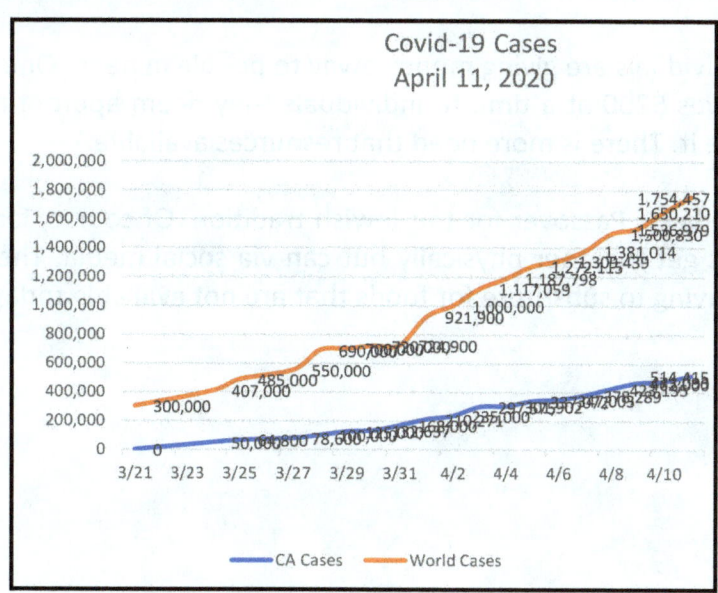

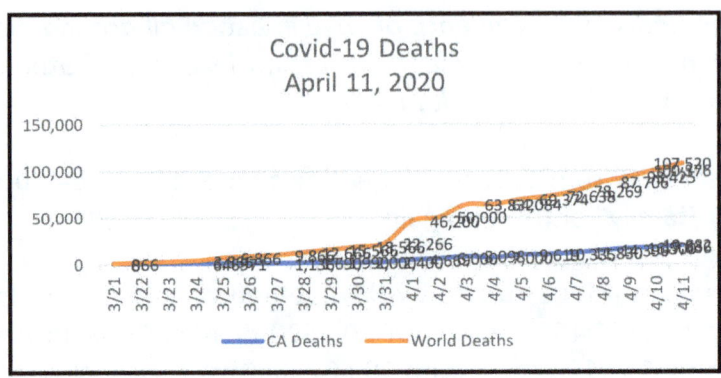

The New York number of cases is flattening but the number of deaths continues to be high ranging from 733 to 799 a day. We need to be cautious in returning to work too soon and causing a new surge in July. It is suggested that we not return to work until we have testing, tracking of cases and treatment. President Trump calls making the decision of when he tells Americans to return to work as "the most important decision of my Presidency." I think he is right about that. One possibility is May 1st but 60% of Americans feel comfortable with that date.

Individuals are giving money away to people in need. One website gives $200 at a time to individuals they deem appropriate to receive it. There is more need that resources available.

Today is Passover for the Jewish tradition. Of course, families cannot get together physically but can via social media. They are also having to substitute for foods that are not available today.

Easter Sunday, April 12, 2020

"SPIRITUAL UNIVERSE – I give up the idea that I belong anywhere other than exactly where I am. I covenant to treat my time in this world as my real and eternal home."

Today I read something is Testimony of Light that seems very appropriate now.

"I sought the Spirit and the Spirit was there all the time.

He came unto His own and His own received Him not.

As I rest now in this Reality I see, with sadness, the truth of these words, I knew Him not. I struggled, fasted, sought for what was already present, perfect and everlasting within me. Like most of us in the body life, I was in illusion; lost in glamour...

But now I let go. I seek for nothing. I absorb and am absorbed by the Spirit of Light, Love, Beauty. I know that I am being remade. Consciousness is expanding to acknowledge and accept the fact of being a Child of the Living Light, of already having, in consciousness all that is needed and reflecting as much of the Spirit as my awareness will permit."
(pp. 106-107)

For me now, there is so much stillness and quiet that it seems a time striving has ceased. I sleep or rest more. There is no sense in rushing as there is nowhere to go. I wonder how many other people are feeling this way. Perhaps that is one of the lessons of this time: to get back to our Spiritual Reality within and without."

Altruism is what is called for now by everyone in the world. We are being ordered but more importantly called to be altruistic at this time of crisis: to put our personal needs above the needs of society. Not everyone is doing this. However, most people are in the U.S. with 97% of the people staying home. I know I am getting restless and so is everyone I talk to. We are tired of being shut in. We are also trying our best to consider the needs of others through money donations, applause for people responding to Covid-19, giving blood, checking on the elderly et cetera. A biproduct of this slowdown economically is a drastic reduction in pollution in the air. This is altruism for the earth itself and the creatures that live on it and in the oceans. I do hope this attitude continues after the pandemic has passed.

Monday, April 13, 2020

"INSPIRATION — I let go and see the evidence of Love in action all around me. The love of the Divine inspires me to express my love for self, others, and for life itself."

I awoke today depressed. Then I turned on the TV to get the good news: the Covid-19 virus curve is flattening in New York and they are planning to lift the stay-at-home order soon. New York is joining other states on the East Coast to have a phased opening of returning to work and life as normal. Thank God!!! Each state will assign a Public Health Officer and an Economic Officer to oversee the transition. It will be guided by science not by desire or politics. Economic recovery will follow on the tails of health recovery. Each state will be in charge of their own plan. Governor Gavin Newsom today also announced a flattening of the curve in California at 23,458 cases and 683 deaths. Tomorrow he will unveil is plan. California is worked with Oregon and Washington on a united response to reopen.

Worldwide today there are 1,872,073 cases and 116,098 deaths. In the U.S. there are 560,891 cases and 22,861 deaths. It hard to fathom the reality that this virus was only identified on January 7, 2020 in Wuhan China. The doctor who discovered it there tried to warn the central government but he was forced by them to retract his statement. The leaders considered the information to be incorrect politically. That doctor died from the disease. When the Chinese people learned of this later on, they were furious with the government. By March 1st there were 1,274 cases in the U.S. and 38 deaths. How rapidly this virus has spread. We would have been in very serious condition had the governments of the world not responded with "stay at home" orders. News programs like PBS Newshour and A Late Show with Stephen Colbert are being filmed from the newscaster's homes as they are now sheltering in place as well.

I also remembered that the best antidote to depression is working out. I hopped on the treadmill then took a hot shower and feel much better. My mood is lifting and the news settles into my consciousness. There IS an end in sight!!!

Tuesday, April 14, 2020

"CONNECTION – I let go and realize that I depend only on the Living Spirit. There is nothing in creation that can separate me from my foundation of trust in the Living Spirit.

Over the weekend there were articles in all major papers criticizing President Trump's handling of the Covid-19 pandemic. He responded in typical fashion by blaming others and saying "he's doing a wonderful job." Specifically, he is blaming the World Heath Organization's response and refusing to send them any more financial support at a time when the world is in the middle of a pandemic. Congress is starting an investigation into this action on his part. Congress is at home now but will return in May 1st.

India has continued its lockdown another two weeks. Italy and Spain are starting to lift some restrictions. What is on everyone's mind is "when will the lockdown ease up?" JPMorgan reported that their profits for the Q1 was down 69%. Clearly our economy is in trouble. However, we cannot ease sanctions until the health problem is solved.

In California Governor Newsom has set up six areas that need to be addressed before restrictions lift.

1. Expand testing and tracking
2. Protect the most vulnerable: seniors, homeless and those with immune disorders.
3. Hospitals and alternative care facilities are stocked with adequate PPE.
4. Engage academia and research in finding therapeutic protocols.
5. Businesses and schools adopt safe practices for social distancing.
6. Continue protecting the general public.

In California today there were 758 total deaths. Worldwide there are 1,945,055 cases with 121,897 deaths. In the U.S. there are 584,072 cases with 23,709 deaths. Cases are levelling off while deaths are increasing. Most people, 80%, have mild symptoms for Covid-19 and recover establishing antibodies in the body. Other, 20% have worse symptoms and/or death. The U.S. 2020 census has been postponed as census takers need to go from door to door to collect data. I answered our census information online about a week ago.

The Governors in the North Easter and Wester states are working together to establish guidelines for a return to "a new normal." President Trump says he has the authority to establish a return date for the country as a whole. Governors are responding by saying "that is not their interpretation of the constitution." How odd, Trump was slow to act, claims "no responsibility for the federal response to the Covid-19 crisis" yet he wants to now take charge? Clearly, he is using his daily news updates as a political rally full of half-truths and ramblings. Some new updates of his last 2 ½ hours! People are starting to not watch them.

Senator Bernie Sanders endorsed Joe Biden for President in 2020 as did former President Barack Obama. The Songs of Comfort website started by Yo-Yo Ma continues to grow on the internet. People are struggling to cope with being in lockdown for now more than a month.

Wednesday, April 15, 2020

"REVITALIZED — I let go and let my heart open to the expression of my natural goodness. I am revitalized by the awareness of my kinship with the Divine. I am excited about the journey I am on.

Eric and I are getting restless. I continue on my routine of exercise, reading, writing, and playing the piano to keep sane. He is less regimented. I encouraged him go on the treadmill after me today. We cannot succumb to negative habits physically or mentally at this time.

Not much new today in the news broadcasts. What is on everyone's mind is "when can we go back to work and recreation." It looks like it will not be before May 1st. Cases worldwide today are 2,008,850 with 129,045 deaths. In the U.S. there are 610,774 cases with 26,119 deaths. The stimulus relief checks from the federal government are going out now. In California Governor Newsom has extended the EDD phone hours to 8:00 a.m. to 8:00 p.m. seven days a week effective Monday the 20th. This is because people were not being able to get through to start their unemployment claims. The time to process such requests in California has gone from the normal three weeks to 24 to 72 hours. People need relief to pay their May rents and mortgages and buy food and medicine. Ten percent of the work force in California is now on unemployment.

Interesting quotes from Testimony of Light:
"Here progress, when made, is always rewarded with service... As one advances to greater light, so one is allowed to teach and guide others of the Group on a lesser path. (p, 125)

Let the perfection of the soul and spirit seep through the window and door of the personality. (pp. 126-127)
We are part of Group Souls — not separate individuals but united. We progress as a group when the least among us has "gotten" the new knowledge to advance the whole.

This then is the message which we want to put across

> (1) There should be no fear of death of the body for it is a gentle passing to a much freer life
> (2) That all life is lived as a serial, that we go from one living to another experience of living at a different rate, i.e., on a higher level of awareness." (p. 129)

Thursday, April 16, 2020

"ONENESS – There is only one Life. That Life is God. That Life is perfect. That Life is my life, now!"

I awoke this morning with fond memories of childhood holidays like Thanksgiving and Christmas. We were all home from school and mom would be fixing a turkey or ham dinner all day long. We would stay in our pajamas reading in the morning then dress for formal dinner together. It was a time of comfort, peace, safety...just the opposite of now. Maybe it is because of reading about Group Souls that I got triggered about the goodness of my childhood. It does seem to be that for the past year I have, in my dreams, been with my family a lot. No one is dead in the dreams even though mom and dad have passed over in real life. Everyone is alive, young, and loving. It is so reassuring.

Reality is hard right now. We are on "stay at home orders" until at least May 1st, another week to go. No one can go out except with a mask now, even babies over two years of age. We cannot return to normal mingling as before until we have tests to identify who has the virus or antibodies for it. We will be checked for our temperatures when we go somewhere to make certain we are not sick. Eric and I were talking yesterday that we think we had the virus in early January. I thought it was the flu but was weak and in bed for two weeks which is highly unusual for me. Then he got it and was sick for about the same amount of time...the time it takes for the virus to go through its process. It is possible that this is so.

I am starting to feel irritable and resigned. There is nothing I can do about the external situation. We are watching a new series on TV called Ozark. It is entertaining. It is an escape from reality for a while. At least we are healthy, safe, have food and warmth during this time. We are so blessed. Still I am restless. I can't wait to be outside again and going to recovery meetings, hugging people and supporting each other. It may be a long time before we feel comfortable hugging each other again. Thank God I have Eric to interact with, talk with, touch. People who live along must be going crazy.

Domestic violence is starting to be a problem now. The hotline for support is shown on the TV. People in two states, Michigan and Ohio, are protesting the "stay at home" order. I'm afraid the next step will be calling out the National Guard. It does not bode well.

Tuesday, April 28, 2020

"HARMONY – I am in harmony with the present moment. The One Life expresses itself through me. I am at peace here and now."

I have disconnected from the news for quite a while because I was getting very depressed. I still stay aware of what is happening in the world but shift my focus above the current circumstances in life to a "higher perspective." I call it "living in the Presence." I wrote more about this in my book My Spiritual Unfolding: Science of Mind. I use mental discipline to live each day with an "expectancy of Good in my life." I felt like I was letting the Covid-19 crisis become my only mental reality. I decided for my sanity I needed to focus on the life I want to cocreate rather than the life as it is now in this world. It takes great mental discipline to do this. Each moment I am aware of my thoughts. If they drift toward the negative ("the virus will never go away, I'll be stuck in the house forever, I'm going crazy") I shift my thinking to the life I want to manifest NOW. I must be patient and thankful for all that I DO have.

I have signed up for another class at the Center for Spiritual Living to start June 11th. It will be on The Varieties of Religious Experience by William James. I ordered the book and have been reading it. It is quite dense and requires concentration. Dr. Kim Kaiser, who teaches the class, is the President of the Holmes Institute where I plan to study this Fall. I obtained two letters of recommendation for the Certificate in Spiritual Education Programs at the Holmes Institute. I then completed my application and sent it in. It is primarily a distance education program so the virus will not cause a problem for classes.

I also took notes on several other spiritual books I mentioned earlier. I cleaned my office and found books by Amit Gaswani on Quantum Physics that are exciting to read. I also cleared away fifty books from my office to make room for the books I will be purchasing for the Certificate in Spiritual Education Program. I also discovered a website about the Abraham Hicks Productions books about the Law of Attraction.

Videos on line are very uplifting and stress focusing on what we want to attract into our lives. There is a video from March 12, 2020 that addressed the situation with Covid-19 specifically that was reassuring.

When I do listen to the news, it is redundant. I've added BBC World News to my watching. One little comment by President Trump will be mulled over all day by the news media. There is continual speculation about when we can move out from "shelter in place" in the U.S. and in the world. Scientists and academicians are working round the clock to find a vaccine for Covid-19. There are many clinical trials in progress worldwide. The one or two that do turn out to work will be mass produced as soon as is humanly possible. In order to be safe, we need to test millions of people a day. In spite of President Trump's proclamation that there is enough testing, the reality is that this is not so. The world will not be back to "normal" until there is a vaccine. Until then, we keep doing our best.

Below are graphs portraying the rise of the Covid-19 cases and deaths worldwide and in the U.S. This reality continues and needs to be coped with as well.

Today there are 1,002,498 cases in the U.S. and 3,083,467 cases in the world.

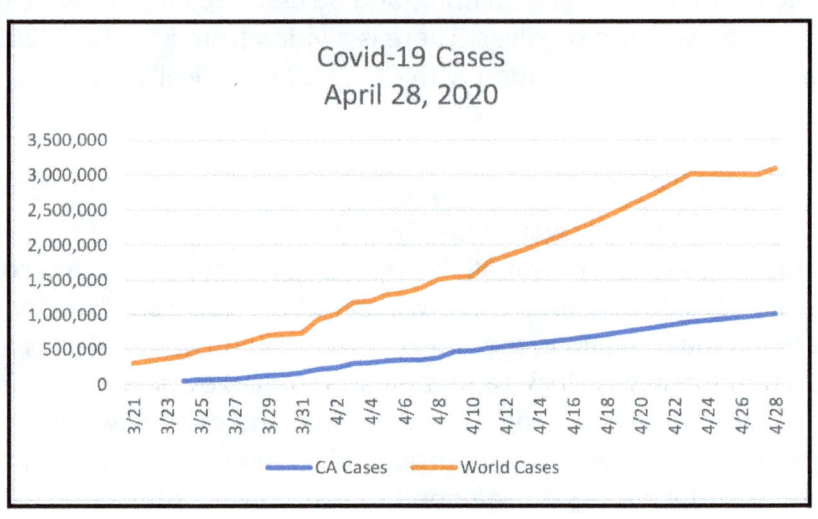

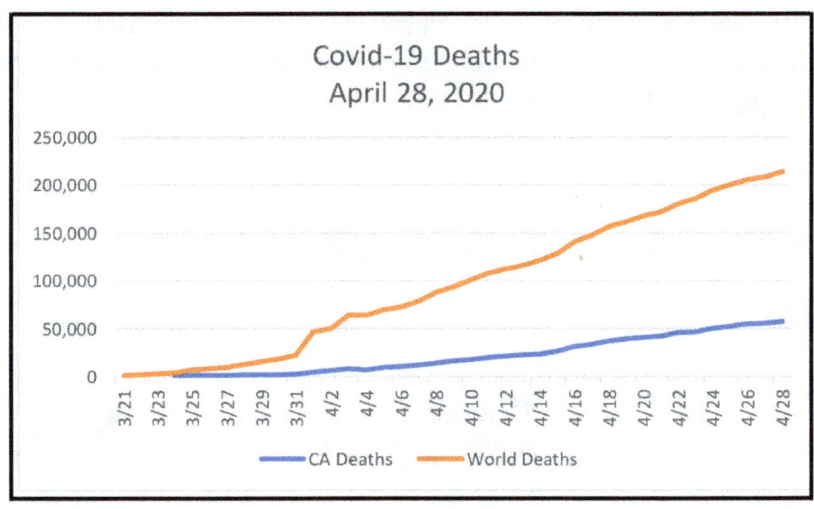

May 12, 2020

"RECOMMITMENT – Today I recommit to being exactly who God created me to be. I am free to give the world the full dose. I am safe to be with. I am as God created."

I noticed today that I have not written since April 28th. This is because my mind has been on others things. As I mentioned on the 28th, I am using discipline to read three to four hours a day. I focus on what IS unfolding for me along the path. What has occurred is publishing My Spiritual Unfolding: Science of Mind. I had TV interview with Bishop O.D. Pringle on May 9th about the book. It will be broadcast later this month.

I will recap the main news topics since April 28th.

- President Trump orders meat packaging plants to reopen. Plants in the Midwest were closed after many workers caughtCovid-19 from the close proximity of their working conditions.
- Remdesivir, by Gilead, was proven to help a patient withCovid-19 in Washington. It is being considered as a possibletreatment for the virus. It is now in clinical trials.
- Men are twice as likely as women to die from the virus.
- On May 1st colleges need to let students know their plans forclasses in the Fall.
- 30 million Americans are out of work and applying forunemployment, 14% of the workforce.
- Airlines now require face masks on flights.
- President Trump offhandedly suggested at his Daily NewsUpdate "if the virus is killed by Clorox maybe we could insertit into humans." This has caused an increase in calls to thenational poison center. Clorox came out the next day sayingunequivocally the produce was not to be injected or injested.

- Europe is opening up slowly.
- J Crew declared bankruptcy.
- The U.S. Supreme Court is hearing cases on phones from their homes. Americans can hear the discussions.
- 33 million American are on unemployment, 15%.
- States in the U.S. are starting to open.

Wednesday, May 13, 2020

"GUIDANCE – All I must do at any moment is to look within to discover that I am guided and inspired by the Presence of Peace. In deepest gratitude, I live my life knowing that I am one with all that is."

I have not written for a while because Covid-19 no longer feels like a crisis. It is a "new way of life." States in the U.S. have been opening up during the past week, some faster than others. Although there are federal guidelines on opening, such as a drop of cases for two weeks before opening, some states are ignoring this recommendation. That is because people are restless and afraid. There are protests by men carrying arms and people shouting at politicians to open the restaurants, hair salons and barber shops, workout clubs and so forth. People are running out of money and need to go back to work. People are afraid and the economic toll is staggering in the U.S. and world over. In the U.S. 36 million people have applied for unemployment bringing it up to 25%. We are witnessing a world economic downfall as never before seen. We will recover, but when is unclear, some predict years. Dr. Fauci at the White House fears that as States open too early, we may experience outbreaks or "hot spots" which will need to be contained. What is needed is clear: testing, contact tracing, quarantining, adequate medical supplies (Personal Protective Equipment) and medical response, and reacting as necessary to the data that emerge. This is true the world over. Some are suggesting using cell phones to trace contacts for those infected with the virus (on a volunteer basis). There is a new development, incidents of early childhood Covid-19 cases. Cases have been reported in several states. Yesterday Prime Minister Johnson of the U.K. stated similar requirements for their citizens (he has recovered from the virus and returned to work).

Schools will most likely continue to be closed this Fall or else have staged class periods so that social distancing can be observed. Colleges will also be closed or turn to distance education models.

Timothy White, Chancellor of the California State University System in California, the largest college system in the U.S., said the CSU is transitioning to distance education for most classes. Today 36 million Americans are out of work, that is one in every four people are not going to work every day. The Covid-19 virus has arrived at the Rohingya Refugee Camps. Prisons are so packed that prisoners have very little protection against infection due to shared ventilation systems and close proximity at food lines. They can only get socially isolated, if infected, by being put into the "hole." The theatres on Broadway in New York and London are still closed and may not recover.

Yesterday I took a friend to the hospital for a surgery that had been postponed due to the virus. I wore a face mask, of course, and had him wear one also and sit in the back seat to try to be six feet apart. This is required in all stores and out in public at large now. When I arrived at the hospital, I was stopped by an attendant who took my temperature and asked about my recent health: had I had a fever, over 104 degrees, diarrhea, fatigue, achiness, shortness of breath and so forth. I said "no" and continued in to pick up my friend.

There is a new normal. It consists of much more consideration for others; appreciation for all those working hard to keep hospitals open, food delivered, online orders deliverers, and medications refilled; and personal sacrifice for the general good. It is drawing out either one's better nature or one's worst nature, both are visible in the world. The website for Songs of Comfort continues to grow with contributions from all types of musicians around the world.

The mental health of everyone is being challenged now. People coming out of comas from the Covid-19 intensive care unit are befuddled and confused. Everyone is tested to the limits. There is a sharp decline in the reports of child abuse in the U.S. probably stemming from the fact that children are not in school to be observed and reported. There is great concern about domestic violence.

The graphs for the spread of the virus from March 21, 2020 until today are below. It appears that the virus is continuing to rise in the world. Today there are 1,372,855 cases in the U.S. and 4,298,269 cases worldwide. There is great concern about what will happen when the virus spreads to Africa and other countries with poor healthcare systems or even worse refugee camps.

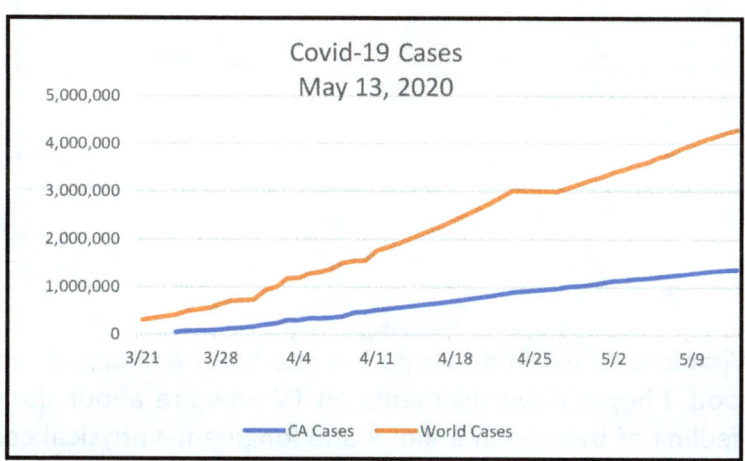

The number of deaths is sobering. In the chart below, we see 82,548 deaths in the U.S. total today and 293,514 deaths worldwide. These numbers are staggering. It is estimated that in the U.S. we will reach 137,000 deaths by the end of the summer. We shall see.

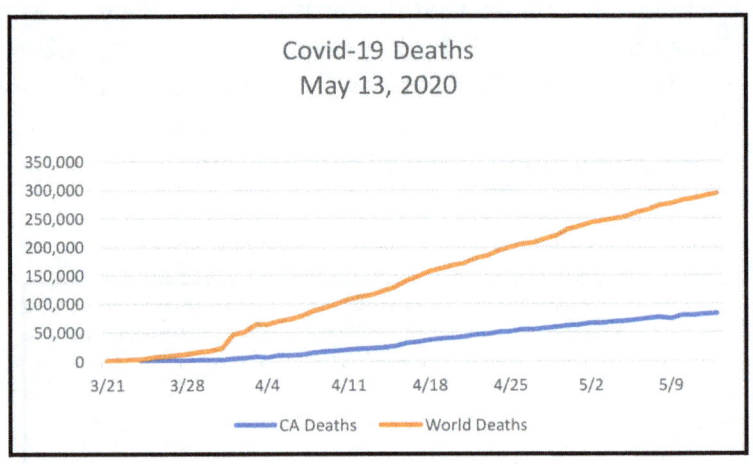

What kind of world do we go out into now? A changed one, for the good, I hope. Advertisements on TV now are about the common feeling of being home alone and longing for physical contact with loved ones. Another common theme is appreciation for everyone working to make our world safe and prosperous again. The upper 1% that controls the world is now having to consider the other 99%, we all need each other from farm workers in the fields providing produce in the markets to CEOs. Everyone needs to stay safe if at all possible. A common sense of shared mission has arisen worldwide. We are one people without borders as far as the virus and its cure are concerned. I believe this is a positive emotional and mental change that will continue to grow as the months and years go by. The world has truly been called to love one another. We must each decide for ourselves how we will respond: with love or fear. We each have different spiritual beliefs and experiences. Let us try to be our best selves as we go forward.

Publishing by: **Maple Leaf Publishing Inc.**

3rd Floor 4915 54 Street
Red Deer, Alberta T4N 2G7, Canada

https://mapleleafpublishinginc.com

To order additional copies of this book, contact:
1-(403)-356-0255

ISBN Paperback: 978 -1 -77419 - 047-0
ISBN eBook: 978 - 1 - 77419 - 048 - 7
Rev. Date: June 08, 2020

www.ingramcontent.com/pod-product-compliance
Lightning Source LLC
Chambersburg PA
CBHW071116030426
42336CB00013BA/2116